8 STEPS
TO
CONQUER CHRONIC PAIN

"I find it helpful to liken your journey to conquer pain to climbing a mountain. I will be your guide in your journey. But it is your journey."

8 STEPS
TO
CONQUER CHRONIC PAIN

A Doctor's Guide to Lifelong Relief

DR. ANDREA FURLAN
MD, PhD, PM&R

For complete cataloguing information, see page 263.

Disclaimer
This book is a general guide only and should never be a substitute for the skill, knowledge, and experience of a qualified medical professional dealing with the facts, circumstances, and symptoms of a particular case.

The nutritional, medical, and health information presented in this book is based on the research, training, and professional experience of the author, and is true and complete to the best of her knowledge. However, this book is intended only as an informative guide for those wishing to know more about health, nutrition, and medicine; it is not intended to replace or countermand the advice given by the reader's personal physician. Because each person and situation is unique, the author and the publisher urge the reader to check with a qualified health-care professional before using any procedure where there is a question as to its appropriateness. A physician should be consulted before beginning any exercise program. The author and the publisher are not responsible for any adverse effects or consequences resulting from the use of the information in this book. It is the responsibility of the reader to consult a physician or other qualified health-care professional regarding his or her personal care.

Design and Production: PageWave Graphics Inc.
Editor: Kathleen Fraser
Indexer: Gillian Watts
Front cover illustration: © Getty Images
Interior illustrations: © Getty Images
Author photo: © Tim Fraser

We acknowledge the support of the Government of Canada.

Canadä

Published by Robert Rose Inc.
120 Eglinton Avenue East, Suite 800, Toronto, Ontario, Canada M4P 1E2
Tel: (416) 322-6552 Fax: (416) 322-6936
www.robertrose.ca

Printed and bound in China

1 2 3 4 5 6 7 8 9 ESP 31 30 29 28 27 26 25 24 23

CONTENTS

Introduction

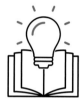

Is This Book for You?

This book is for anyone with chronic pain. Medical specialists define chronic pain as pain lasting more than three months. It could be pain that persists after an injury has healed, a condition that has been treated or even pain without a known cause. You may see yourself in some of the cases that I describe in this book. I will explain that not all chronic pain is the same. You may not need to use all strategies in this book, but I hope you will find some things you can change, start or stop doing that will help you to gain a better quality of life.

This book is not medical advice

This book will give you knowledge. I hope you can use this knowledge to discuss with your own healthcare provider what the best strategy is for you. Only your doctor or therapist knows your situation. They have all the important details of your medical history and they can examine you and order diagnostic tests. Check the disclaimer of this book on page 4 for more information.

What Does It Mean to Conquer Pain?

Let me start this book at the ending.

Conquering pain is different for each person. What does it mean to you? Take a moment to think about what you want to do about your pain. What do you imagine your future will be?

For some people, conquering pain means the pain disappears completely and for good. For others, it simply means a better quality of life.

You may have already tried a variety of treatments to eliminate your pain. Perhaps you have seen many specialists and therapists, invested time and spent money, and you are still in pain. Maybe your pain will disappear with the strategies that I explain in this book. Or maybe not, but it is possible you will have a better quality of life.

TO MAKE A CHANGE, DO SOMETHING DIFFERENT
What prompted you to pick up this book? You probably chose this book because you want a change.

If you want something to change in your life, you need to start doing something different today. If you don't start doing anything different today, chances are that your pain will not be different tomorrow. If you postpone making changes in your life, you have already made a decision to remain the same.

Take a moment to think about what it is that you are searching for.

What Is Your Pain Story?

Pain is not the same for everyone. I have never seen two individuals with exactly the same pain presentation.

Are you uncertain about your diagnosis? Are you concerned about your future? Are you confused because there seem to be so many treatments available? Are you worried because you have not tried all the options yet?

Maybe you don't believe that your doctor knows how to treat your pain. You have had this pain for so long and your doctor still doesn't know the cause. Why not? You've looked on the Internet and found so many web sites, blogs, videos, podcasts, newsletters, books, vitamins and exercises, and you are confused. You don't know where to go or who to trust anymore.

How many doctors or therapists have you seen in your life for your pain problem? How many hours of physiotherapy, manual therapy and counseling?

SEARCHING FOR A QUICK CURE

Some people with chronic pain are on a journey to find a specialist who has the cure for their pain. They think they will find a professional who will tell them exactly where the pain is coming from and will eliminate that pain in a few seconds. Let me tell you, that is very unlikely.

How many radiological exams have you had? I have seen patients who had hundreds of X-rays, dozens of CT scans and a handful of MRIs. The problem is that there is always something that appears abnormal on these exams. It is almost impossible to find any person who has a completely normal radiological exam.

How many injections, nerve blocks or surgeries have you had? My record was a patient who had 54 surgeries on her abdomen to try to eliminate her chronic abdominal pain.

How many pills have you ingested in your life to try to eliminate this pain? If you could add all the pills that you've taken, how many would that be? My record was a patient who was taking 192 tablets per day. Almost a cereal bowl full of pills.

Some people take desperate measures to get rid of chronic pain. I had a patient who had excruciating low back pain. He took a scalpel and, using a mirror, tried to do surgery on himself. He ended up in the emergency department and was left with a terrible scar. Fortunately, he did not cause any injury to his spinal cord, or he would have become paraplegic.

In my experience, the most tragic cases are when a patient requests medical assistance to terminate their life because they can't endure the pain anymore.

Knowledge Is Power

This book is a compilation of my 30 years of experience as a pain physician and scientist. It contains the information that I give to my patients who are suffering from chronic pain. I hope this book will give you hope.

I believe that having the right knowledge gives you the power to transform your life. A person who understands what is happening to their body and mind is empowered to discuss diagnoses and therapeutic options. Fear makes our bodies release stress hormones that aggravate pain, but a person with adequate knowledge is less fearful. And those who have knowledge are more inclined to agree to and stick with interventions that work for them.

> This book will give you knowledge, and knowledge gives you the power to conquer your pain.

CONNECT WITH ME ON SOCIAL MEDIA

I would love to know what you are doing when you read this book.

If you want to connect with me and tell me what you like (or didn't like) about this book, tag me on social media using the hashtag #ConquerPainWithDrFurlan.

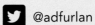 @adfurlan

dr.andrea.furlan

dr.andrea.furlan

WATCH ME ON YOUTUBE
https://www.youtube.com/c/DrAndreaFurlan

You will find QR codes throughout this book that link to specific videos on my channel.

VISIT MY CHANNEL

FREE WORKSHEETS
If you would like to receive and print at home the exercises included in this book plus many more worksheets, go to www.doctorandreafurlan.com.

#ConquerPainWithDrFurlan

Your Journey through the Eight Steps

The chapters in this book follow a progressive structure that leads you on an eight-step journey to conquer pain. You will get the most out of this book if you read the steps in sequence.

Your Journey

I find it helpful to liken your journey to conquer pain to climbing a mountain. I will be your guide in your journey. But it is your journey. I cannot climb the mountain for you or with you. I will provide you with the knowledge, tools and resources. I will share with you what I have learned from many other patients, from colleagues and from the latest scientific research.

Your journey starts before you arrive at the base of the mountain. Depending on the type of mountain, you will need to learn about hiking, mountaineering, rock climbing, alpine or ice climbing. You should read guides, watch videos and talk to other people who have done this.

Once you understand what you need to help you along the way, you must visit a specialized store and purchase the necessary equipment. You will need to pack food for many weeks or months.

What Are the Eight Steps?

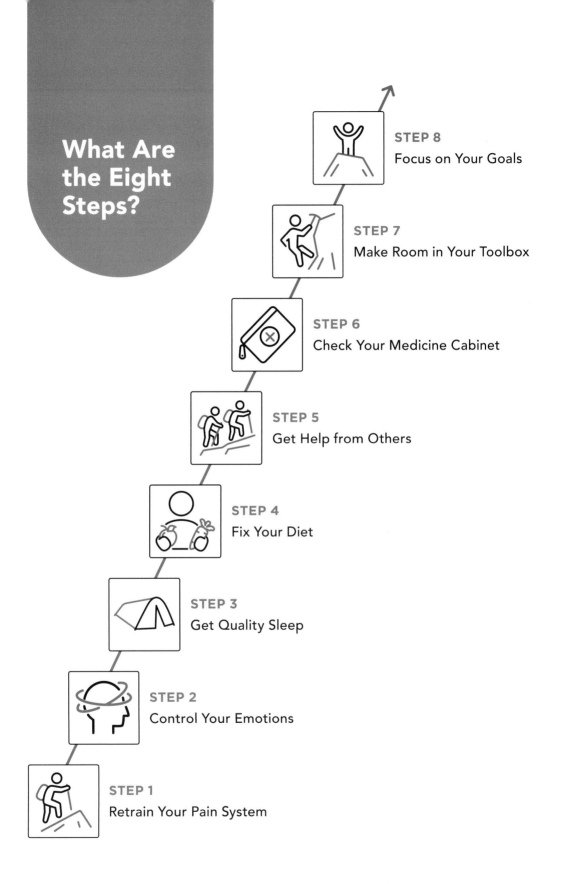

STEP 8
Focus on Your Goals

STEP 7
Make Room in Your Toolbox

STEP 6
Check Your Medicine Cabinet

STEP 5
Get Help from Others

STEP 4
Fix Your Diet

STEP 3
Get Quality Sleep

STEP 2
Control Your Emotions

STEP 1
Retrain Your Pain System

You need to be sure your fitness levels are adequate for the altitude you will climb, or you could develop mountain sickness or experience shortness of breath. You should be physically and mentally prepared for potential challenges, such as falling rocks, rain and snow, heat during the day and cold nights, as well as your physiological needs.

Maybe you are bringing someone with you to the mountain or maybe or you will meet your group there. Together you will decide how to work to reach your goals.

Finally, after months of preparation, you will be ready for your first steps up. Each person will travel at a different speed on their own trail; you will find the one that works best for you.

WE DON'T CHOOSE PAIN; PAIN CHOOSES US

A climbing journey has some similarities to conquering chronic pain, but also differences. While mountain climbing is optional, chronic pain is not a choice. No one wakes up one morning and says, "I need a challenge, so I will inflict pain on my body and then I will overcome it."

Pain happens as an injury, an accident or a disease. Sometimes it appears without an apparent cause, as with a neuropathy (damage to the nerves) or fibromyalgia. We don't choose pain; pain chooses us.

What is the first obstacle that I see in many of my patients? They deny chronic pain. They don't see the mountain in front of them. And I can't guide them to climb it if they don't believe they have chronic pain.

"Each person will travel at a different speed on their own trail; you will find the one that works best for you."

Are you ready for your journey?

Here's our itinerary:

WHAT IS PAIN?

In *What Is Pain?* we will examine what pain actually is.

Our body has a pain system that acts like the alarm system of a house. When the pain system is working well, pain is a sensation that alerts our brain that something needs to be fixed or eliminated. However, there might be malfunctioning of the pain system itself, leading to false alarms, increased pain volume or short circuits in the brain. They prolong the pain without an injury or disease triggering it. In this chapter:

- We will learn about the three kinds of pain: nociceptive, neuropathic and nociplastic. Basically, nociceptive pain occurs when the alarm system is working well, while neuropathic pain occurs when there is an injury or disease in the pain system, and nociplastic pain occurs because the pain system is intact but malfunctioning.
- When the alarm system of the house malfunctions, we need to fix the alarm system instead of trying to find a fire to put out. Much chronic pain is caused by abnormal pain systems, so we need to learn how to fix the pain system instead of trying to find where the injury causing the pain is.

GETTING A DIAGNOSIS

Next, in *Getting a Diagnosis,* we will visit a pain clinic and learn how a doctor diagnoses chronic pain.

- We will talk about the types of doctors that treat patients with chronic pain, including pain clinics and specialists, and what the doctors will ask you, which tests they might run and why labs and images aren't always necessary.
- Often, a physical examination is all the doctor needs. We will also look at some messages that doctors give their patients and how they can be planting the seeds of pain.

- We consider why some people, including those who have had adverse childhood experiences, are more likely to have chronic pain.
- We will also introduce the toolbox, which includes many tools for you to use when you have chronic pain.

1   STEP 1: RETRAIN YOUR PAIN SYSTEM

In *Step 1: Retrain Your Pain System,* you will be introduced to strategies to retrain a malfunctioning pain system.

I will explain how it is possible to fix the pain system without medication, injections or surgery. Think of it as physiotherapy for your brain. Fixing the pain system does not require expensive equipment or therapy sessions. Fixing the pain system does require that you come with an open mind, receptive to new and exciting mind-body exercises.

Key points in this chapter include:

- The pain system functions to protect us from danger and preserve our body's integrity. But when the pain system is malfunctioning, this overprotection keeps us from fully living our lives.
- The pain system is not just in the brain. It involves the neurological, emotional, immunological and endocrinological systems.

I use an integrative pain medicine approach that treats the individual as a whole. While everyone else is trying to treat my patient's pain, I am trying to treat the person who has the pain.

2   STEP 2: CONTROL YOUR EMOTIONS

In *Step 2: Control Your Emotions,* you will see how your emotions affect your pain.

Most people with chronic pain acknowledge that pain affects their emotions. Many feel depressed because they are in pain all the time. They are more anxious about their future because they think it will just keep getting worse.

However, the reverse is also true. Your emotions can affect your pain. But few people with chronic pain acknowledge that their state of mind affects their pain. We will learn that:

- The pain system shares a lot of neuronal, hormonal and immunological pathways with the emotional system.
- Pain can be initiated, aggravated or maintained by emotions, thoughts and memories.
- The pain system is influenced by our previous experiences, especially from childhood, and by the social environment, our relationships and spiritual conditions.
- There is a strong connection between mind and body.

> Our body can express our emotions, and pain is a very common way in which emotions are expressed.

 3 **STEP 3:
GET QUALITY SLEEP**

Step 3: Get Quality Sleep **is all about recharging your batteries.**

Sleep is an important part of our lives, especially in people with chronic pain. Few people take sleep seriously, and even fewer take action to ensure they have a good quality of sleep. Most people would agree that chronic pain causes poor sleep, but what many don't know is that poor sleep also causes chronic pain. In this chapter, we will talk about:

- The relationship between chronic pain and poor sleep
- How to improve sleep efficiency without medications

 4 **STEP 4:
FIX YOUR DIET**

Step 4: Fix Your Diet **is about nutrition and healthy, mindful eating.**

I have seen many people who suffer from chronic pain because they are malnourished and lack essential nutrients such as vitamins, minerals, proteins, energy and essential fats. In this chapter, we will examine:

- How many people eat for the wrong reasons. In our culture, we eat what is quick, affordable and easy. We eat to comfort our anxiety, disappointments and loneliness.
- Mindful eating and how you can transform your meals into nourishment for your body, mind and soul

- The anti-inflammatory diet that I recommend to all my patients with chronic inflammation
- Why it is hard for people with chronic pain to maintain a healthy diet

5 STEP 5: GET HELP FROM OTHERS

In *Step 5: Get Help from Others,* we learn how to communicate with the people around us.

Chronic pain is invisible. People cannot see your pain, and there is no way to prove that you are in pain. People with chronic pain tell me that they would prefer to have an amputation, cancer or a cardiac disease, so at least people would believe them and feel empathy for them. Unfortunately, people with chronic pain are misinterpreted as lazy, drug-seeking, unreliable and "difficult." Many physicians refuse to accept people with chronic pain in their family medicine practices because they are too "complex."

Conquering pain is a team effort. Yet many people with chronic pain lack the skills to communicate with their family, friends and coworkers and even with their doctor. We will discuss:

- How to explain your pain to your doctor
- Talking about your pain to your partner, family, friends and coworkers
- The many resources that are available to people with chronic pain, such as pain clinics and peer-support groups

6 STEP 6: CHECK YOUR MEDICINE CABINET

In *Step 6: Check Your Medicine Cabinet,* we look at various medications.

Not all types of chronic pain respond well to painkillers. Depending on the type of pain, the medications can either help or make the pain worse. In medical school, we learn a lot about medications, and that is why medical doctors like to use them. In this chapter, we will look at:

- How the types of medications we use to treat chronic pain are different than the ones we use to treat acute pain from an injury or inflammation. These include antidepressants and antiepileptics.

- Opioids and other painkillers. The name suggests they kill the pain; this may be true for some kinds of pain but not others.
- Options such as injections, topical creams, cannabis-based compounds, and over-the-counter medications that do not need a doctor's prescription

7 STEP 7: MAKE ROOM IN YOUR TOOLBOX

In *Step 7: Make Room in Your Toolbox,* we discuss other options to manage pain.

The place where you go to find ways to conquer chronic pain is your toolbox. Drugs are only one tool in this toolbox. We will discuss the 5M toolbox:

- Movement as a therapeutic intervention to treat chronic pain and fix the malfunctioning pain system
- Mind-body interventions such as mindfulness, meditation, hypnosis and relaxation
- Manual therapies that you can do yourself at home
- Modalities such as heat, cold and electrotherapy
- Medications, including anti-inflammatory, analgesics, muscle relaxants, opioids and cannabis-based compounds

8 STEP 8: FOCUS ON YOUR GOALS

In *Step 8: Focus on Your Goals,* you will see how you can conquer pain step by step by setting goals.

In this chapter, I will show you "the pain trajectory," or the course that pain may take in the lifetime of a person. We'll look at strategies to change that trajectory.

We will discuss how you can create goals for yourself in your journey to conquer pain. In my experience, patients who conquered their pain are the ones who had a clear path of specific, measurable, attainable, relevant, time-bound, evaluable and revisable (SMARTer) goals. This will avoid disappointments and frustrations.

Once you reach your goals, you will be able to say you have conquered your chronic pain.

Record Your Journey

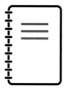

Today, starting now, get a notebook and begin a journal with me. Here are some questions to get you going on your journey. I will ask you to reflect on these questions again at the end of the book. It's important to keep a record so you can track your progress.

Write down what you are thinking today, date your answers and then compare your answers when you finish this book.

1 Do you know everything you need to know about your pain?

2 Have you explored all the possibilities to eliminate this pain?

3 If you must live with this pain for the rest of your life, do you think you have all the tools in your toolbox to move on and live your life to the full potential?

4 Is there anything you want to achieve in life, but chronic pain is in the way?

5 How would you measure your own success — your victory over pain?

If you want to find the answers to these questions, keep reading this book.

NOTE

Throughout this book, I will mention some of the patients I have treated over the past 30 years of my practice as a pain specialist. The cases have been slightly modified and their names have been changed to protect their privacy and confidentiality.

"It's important to keep a record so you can track your progress."

My journey to conquer
chronic pain starts today.
I am motivated to learn new
strategies and I am committed
to making the necessary changes.
I will look up to other people
who have done this. I will
read this book and I will
complete the exercises.

What Is Pain?

In this chapter, we look at what pain is and how it functions as an alarm system for our bodies. Then we explore the different kinds of pain. It is important for you to understand this before you begin your climb up the mountain.

What Pain Is Not

Pain is not an accurate measure of how much damage there is in any part of the body. There is no correlation between pain intensity and degree of harm.

Let me say that again, just in case you think you didn't read it correctly.

- A person can have no chest pain and be dying of a heart attack (a serious harm).
- A person may have a massive stroke (serious harm) and not feel any headache.
- A person may have advanced ovarian cancer (serious harm) and not have any pain at all.
- A person may have an amputated leg and feel excruciating pain on the non-existent foot (no serious harm). If the foot doesn't exist, then the pain is clearly not a sign that the foot is being harmed.
- A person may feel severe pain by imagining an object piercing their skin when, in fact, there is nothing touching their skin. I will show you a case where this actually happened.

Everyone Experiences Pain Differently

The experience of pain is variable between men and women. Men have a higher threshold for pain than women. There are also genetic and environmental factors that influence how much pain each person perceives. When romantic couples were tested in the laboratory, they reported experiencing less pain when they were holding hands than when they were tested separately from each other.

People with previous memories of pain are more sensitive to pain. Studies have shown that babies born prematurely who were exposed to painful procedures in the neonatal care unit had a higher incidence of chronic pain as adults.

Children of people with chronic pain tend to have a lower threshold to painful stimuli. That means it takes less stimulation to make them feel pain. They also develop more chronic pain as adults. The explanation may be more than genetics; it can also come from their learning environment and a normalization of feeling and expressing pain.

People with certain personality traits and emotions are also more prone to suffering than other people from the same stimulus. These include pessimistic thoughts, perfectionism, people-pleasing, a sense of perceived injustice and low self-esteem. Emotions such as sadness, frustration and anger can also influence how much pain we feel. When the person learns how to manage their personality traits and their emotions, their pain levels can drop a lot.

We'll talk more about these differences when we discuss your pain system.

> There is no correlation between pain intensity and degree of harm. Recent advances in neuroscience have helped us to understand that the amount of pain we feel is not a good measure of how much injury or disease is affecting our body.

Why do I have pain all the time and all over my body?

There is a condition called fibromyalgia, in which a person feels pain all the time and in many parts of their body. With fibromyalgia, the pain system is malfunctioning. Ask your doctor if you have fibromyalgia. Throughout this book we will be talking more about fibromyalgia and exploring strategies to retrain the pain system and reduce its impact on your quality of life.

The Pain System

Our body is formed of many systems. You may be familiar with the digestive, respiratory, reproductive, cardiovascular, neurological and immunological systems.

Did you know that we have a pain system? The pain system is made up of sensors all over our body that are on the alert to detect danger. These sensors send impulses via the nerves, and they enter the spinal cord, where they connect to neurons that will activate the various pain centers in the brain. The function of the pain system is to alert us that there is some danger to ourselves.

The function of the pain system

The biology of the pain system begins with the function of pain.

The function of pain is to protect us from injuries and diseases by alerting the mind that there is some danger and it needs to be removed.

THE BOTTOM-UP PAIN ACTIVATING PATHWAYS

To fulfill its function, the pain system has sensors distributed all over, mostly in the skin, but also in the bones, tendons, muscles, organs, veins, arteries and some membranes, like the meninges that protect the brain. It is interesting that the brain itself does not have pain sensors, or receptors.

When these pain receptors, also known as **nociceptors**, are activated by something too hot or cold, or too much pressure or inflammation, that will trigger an electrical impulse. The impulse travels through the peripheral nerves and enters the central nervous system, either in the spinal cord or the brain stem, where they can be modulated. Then, another connection (we call this a synapse) is made with a second neuron that will transmit the message to the brain. This process is known as **nociception**.

> *Modulation* is like the volume dial in your radio. Pain modulation means your body can increase or decrease the intensity of the pain sensation.

When the electrical impulse arrives at the brain

The electrical impulse, sent from neuron to neuron, will activate various regions in the brain. There is no single area of the brain that is responsible for pain. Unlike other sensations, like vision and hearing, which have dedicated areas of the brain just for these functions, pain does not have a single area.

The centers of pain in the brain are formed by a network of neurons and connections in the brain linked to perception

THE BOTTOM-UP PAIN ACTIVATING PATHWAYS

1 Sensors for danger

2 Peripheral nerves

3 Spinal cord (for nerves arriving from the body) or brain stem (for nerves arriving from the head)

4 Thalamus

5 Amygdala

6 Cerebellum

7 Somatosensory cortex (S1)

8 Sensory cortex (S2)

9 Insula

10 Anterior cingulate cortex (ACC)

11 Prefrontal cortex (PFC)

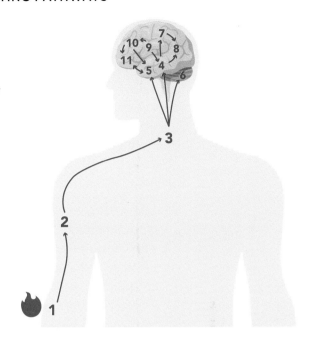

The bottom-up pain activating pathways respond to any stimulus perceived as dangerous (hot, cold, pressure, inflammation). Nerves transmit this sensation as an electrical impulse from the damaged area to the central nervous system (the spinal cord). The spinal cord modulates the sensation and delivers it to the brain, where a network of neurons and links connected to the perception of pain are activated.

of pain, and these brain areas are activated when you experience a sensation that is perceived as dangerous.

These various areas of the brain and brain stem are integrated, and scientists can see them using specific brain imaging studies in the laboratory. We observe these areas lighting up when the person feels pain, imagines pain, remembers pain or is seeing someone else suffering pain (empathy).

Each person activates different areas for the same painful stimulation. Even the same person will activate different areas at different times, sometimes even on the same day. This variation is what makes pain a complex phenomenon to study and to treat.

It is interesting to see how the same person responds differently to the same painful stimulation. If the stimulation occurs when the person feels safe and happy, they will activate (or not activate) some areas of the pain centers, but if they feel threatened and sad, they will activate (or not activate) other areas. The brain areas are also activated differently if the pain is acute (as in the first time the person is feeling that sensation) or if the pain is chronic (as in the case of someone who has persistent low back pain).

These discoveries have been made possible in the past 20 years by advances in brain imaging techniques (Davis, Flor, Greely et al., 2017).

Many different areas of the brain react to pain

These are some of the primary areas of the brain that are activated when there is an acute pain stimulus:

- **SOMATOSENSORY CORTEX:** gives the precise localization of the stimulus
- **AMYGDALA:** fear, worry, anticipation
- **INSULA:** information processing, emotional and cognitive components of pain
- **THALAMUS:** relay center
- **HYPOTHALAMUS:** stress response (fight, flight, or freeze)
- **PREMOTOR CORTEX:** planning for movement
- **MOTOR CORTEX:** movement; activation of muscles to move a body part
- **CINGULATE CORTEX:** concentration, focus
- **PREFRONTAL CORTEX:** problem-solving, meaning, explanation, interpretation, memory
- **CEREBELLUM:** movement, coordination and cognition
- **HIPPOCAMPUS:** memory
- **BRAIN STEM:** relaying information from the brain and activating the top-down pathways

The ***periaquedutal gray*** (PAG) and ***rostral ventromedial medulla*** (RVM) are areas of the brain stem controlled by the brain above it. The PAG and RVM are important areas of the top-down pain inhibitory pathways, as it is here where the endogenous, or internal, opioids and endogenous cannabinoids are produced.

THE TOP-DOWN PAIN INHIBITORY PATHWAYS

Once the brain is aware of the message signaling danger, it begins a process of turning off the alarm signals coming from the periphery. It starts within certain areas of the brain, in the anterior cingulate cortex, the prefrontal cortex, the insula and the amygdala. These areas activate the periaqueductal gray (PAG) and the rostral ventral medulla (RVM) in the brain stem. Then, the RVM activates the

THE TOP-DOWN PAIN INHIBITORY PATHWAYS

1 Anterior cingulate cortex (ACC)

2 Prefrontal cortex (PFC)

3 Insula

4 Amygdala

5 Periaqueductal gray (PAG)

6 Rostral ventromedial medulla (RVM)

7 Spinal cord

8 Periphery

opiods + cannabinoids

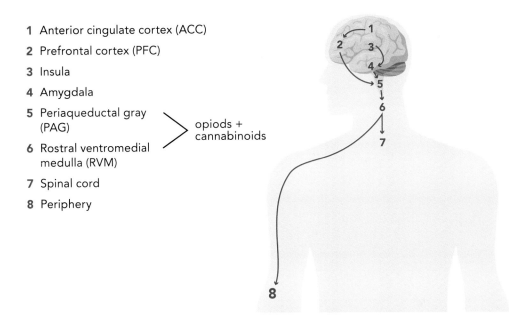

The top-down pain inhibitory pathways start with areas of the brain being activated, and they send commands to the brain stem (where the PAG and RVM are located) to release powerful analgesic substances that will be transported to the spinal cord and to the periphery to stop these painful sensations.

endogenous, or internal, opiod system to release endorphins, dynorphins and enkephalins. These are potent opioids and they will block the pain at various levels: the brain, the spinal cord and, in some organs, such as the kidneys and the heart.

The brain stem is our internal pharmacy, in that it can produce and release our own opioids and cannabinoids very quickly on demand. (We discuss this subject more in *Step 6: Check Your Medicine Cabinet.*) In some chronic pain populations, this internal pharmacy is deficient and is not operating normally, which is the case with fibromyalgia.

MAPPING THE PAIN

The *somatosensory area of the brain* will indicate where the danger is. Our skin is very well mapped in the brain: for every inch of skin, there are a lot of sensors. This makes the skin map in the brain very precise. But the mapping is not so precise for other organs.

Let me give you an example. If you pinch the skin around your mouth or your fingers with a toothpick, even with your eyes closed, your brain will inform you exactly where the toothpick is pricking you. That is because the skin around the mouth and the tips of the fingers is very precisely mapped. For other areas of the skin, however, like the back of the thigh, the mapping is less precise.

Yet the skin is much more accurate at mapping than the internal organs. Take the heart, for example. If a person is having a heart attack, they will not be able to say, "I'm having a myocardial infarct in the left-inferior side of my heart, or the upper right corner of the heart." The heart, like any other internal organ, is not well mapped in the brain.

When there is pain originating from the stomach, gallbladder, ureters, bowels, uterus or muscles, the brain will not be able to localize exactly where the problem is. A person with appendicitis may have pain in the lower right side of their abdomen, but often they will feel pain in the middle of the abdomen, the lower back, the hip or the upper right side of the abdomen.

YES, THERE IS A PAIN SYSTEM

Children learn in biology classes in middle school about the various systems that compose the human body. But the pain system is not included in the curriculum.

Even though 100 percent of people experience pain and 20 percent of people will end up developing chronic pain in their lifetime, most will have no idea what pain is. Or worse, they have the wrong idea of what pain is.

DANGER OR NO DANGER?

The **autonomic nervous system** is part of the peripheral nerve system and it is formed by the **sympathetic** and the **parasympathetic nervous systems.**

- The sympathetic nervous system is responsible for the fight, flight or freeze response. It is activated in stressful situations and it is essential for our survival when there is danger.
- The parasympathetic nervous system is the opposite. It is activated when we are not in a dangerous situation. We call it the rest, digest and recover system.

Other brain areas that are activated are involved in the interpretation of the sensory stimulus. They are related to emotions, attention, memory, anticipation, expectation, interpretation and meaning. They are activated when we feel pain, when we remember pain, when we imagine pain or when we see someone in pain. How much these other areas are activated will depend on how much the brain judges the pain as a threat. When there is a perception that the pain signals are very dangerous, it doesn't matter whether the area is small or large. If there is a perception of danger, the brain may activate all of the areas that are involved in the suffering and emotional aspect of pain.

There are other factors that also interfere with the perception of pain. These include paying attention to the sensation or getting distracted, having empathetic people around you or being alone, or having a good day and feeling happy as opposed to having a bad day and being in a bad mood. Pain is an opinion about what is happening in the body, and the brain will try to get as much information as possible to interpret the sensation. Is it dangerous or not? Should I stay or should I leave immediately?

ACTIVATING THE PAIN SYSTEM
A tiny area of damage can activate the whole pain system, including the areas of emotions, if the brain perceives that sensation as a danger. There are situations in which the brain will not perceive a great danger, but it will still activate large areas of the pain system, because there is anticipation, or an expectation, that the pain will be very intense.

"Some brain areas that interpret sensory stimulus are related to emotions, attention, memory, anticipation, expectation, interpretation and meaning. They are activated when we feel pain, when we remember pain, when we imagine pain or when we see someone in pain."

Three Kinds of Pain

How the three kinds of pain set off alarms in our brain

There are basically three kinds of pain: *nociceptive, neuropathic* and *nociplastic.* I wish I had less technical terms to use here, but unfortunately, I don't.

Pain can be compared to an alarm system of a house. In a house, the alarm will sound when there is an intruder, water leak or smoke.

It is good that we have an alarm system for our body; otherwise, we could be damaging our body and not even realize it.

NOCICEPTIVE PAIN

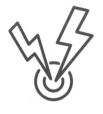

Nociceptive pain occurs when there is an injury or disease such as a fractured bone, appendicitis or inflammatory arthritis. The pain system will do what it is supposed to do. It will alert the brain to do something about it. The person has to stop what they are doing and seek medical care immediately. Once the person receives proper treatment, the pain system doesn't need to continue to be active, so it will deactivate itself. The injury heals or the disease is treated, and the alarm system becomes silent.

NEUROPATHIC PAIN

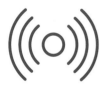

Neuropathic pain occurs when there is an injury or illness to the nerve system itself. It is similar to a situation where the wires of the alarm system have been cut or there is a short circuit in the system. Examples of this kind of pain are after a stroke, spinal cord injury, multiple sclerosis, shingles or nerve pain caused by diabetes.

NOCIPLASTIC PAIN

Nociplastic pain means the injury has healed or the disease has been treated and the wires are intact, but the alarm system is malfunctioning. The pain volume might be too loud (the person feels pain more intensely) or there are spontaneous false alarms. When pain lasts longer than the expected healing period, that means that the pain system has become sensitized or some modifications have occurred in how the pain is being processed. In this situation, the alarm system continues to alert the person beyond the healing period. Nociplastic pain is a kind of **chronic pain.** It can start as nociceptive pain, neuropathic pain or both. (See the following pages for more about chronic pain.)

> **Nociceptive pain** occurs when the alarm system is working well, **neuropathic pain** is when the wires are damaged, and **nociplastic pain** mean the alarm system is malfunctioning.
>
> You will want to remember the term **nociplastic**, because we talk a lot about it in this book. In medical terms, "noci" means pain or injury and "plastic" means capable of being shaped or formed.

What does it feel like? Characteristics of the three kinds of pain

We've seen how the three kinds of pain alert our pain system. In some patients, these three kinds of pain occur simultaneously. All three kinds of pain are real. The person is not fabricating, imagining or inventing pain. They feel pain. But each of these kinds of pain has distinct characteristics.

See pages 54–55 in *Getting a Diagnosis* to learn how pain specialists diagnose different kinds of pain.

NOCICEPTIVE PAIN

- *Nociceptive pain* is usually acute, sharp and can be precisely located when it happens around the skin, bones or tendons.
- Nociceptive pain from internal organs is hard to localize and may "refer" to another area. (**Referred pain** is pain that you perceive at a site other than the place of origin.) An example is menstrual cramps, where the pain may be referred to the inner thighs, lower back and pelvic area.

NEUROPATHIC PAIN

- *Neuropathic pain* is described as burning, tingling, electrical shocks, throbbing, piercing and numbing. Examples include post-herpetic neuralgia, trigeminal neuralgia and diabetic neuropathy.
- Some injuries to the central and peripheral nerve systems may lead to neuropathic pain, such as stroke, brain injury and multiple sclerosis.
- Compression of peripheral nerves can also cause neuropathic pain, such as carpal tunnel syndrome and radiculopathy.

WHAT IS PAIN? **29**

NOCIPLASTIC PAIN

- *Nociplastic pain* is characterized by diffuse, hard to locate, constant pain. There is no position that will alleviate the pain. Examples are migraine, tension-type headache, temporomandibular joint (TMJ) dysfunction, irritable bowel syndrome, chronic pelvic pain, painful bladder and fibromyalgia.
- As noted, nociplastic pain can occur in combination with the other two kinds of pain.

Acute Pain Versus Chronic Pain

Acute pain is pain that lasts less than three months.

Chronic pain is ongoing continuous pain that last for three months or longer and has passed the expected healing period.

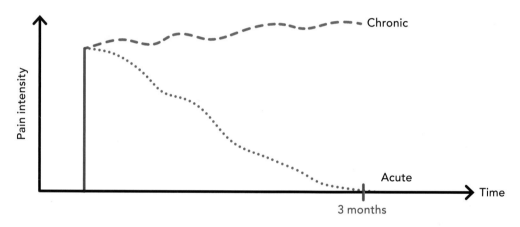

Chronic pain affects the person's ability to think, to concentrate and to plan. People who suffer chronic pain often struggle to find the motivation they need to overcome that pain. This is very different from an athlete who is fit and mentally strong who decides they want to climb a mountain. People with chronic pain are usually tired, depressed, anxious and frustrated. It is hard for them to find the energy to defeat the enemy because they carry a heavy burden of pain 24 hours a day. Because pain never leaves them, they feel defeated already.

CHRONIC PRIMARY PAIN VERSUS CHRONIC SECONDARY PAIN

Another way to classify pain is by dividing it into primary and secondary pain. Some people prefer this classification system because it has been included in the 11th Revision of the International Classification of Diseases (ICD) and is distributed worldwide by the World Health Organization.

Chronic pain can be primary or secondary:

- Chronic primary pain represents chronic pain as a disease itself.

- Chronic secondary pain is chronic pain where the pain is a symptom of an underlying condition.

These are examples of chronic primary pain:

- Fibromyalgia: widespread pain, sleep disturbances, low mood and fatigue

- Complex regional pain syndrome (CRPS): usually affects the limbs – an arm, leg, hand or foot – but can affect any part of your body

- Chronic migraine

- Temporomandibular joint disorder (TMJ): jaw and facial pain

- Irritable bowel syndrome

- Nonspecific low back pain

These are examples of chronic secondary pain:

- Post-herpetic neuralgia: a painful complication of shingles

- Chronic pain after a spinal cord injury

- Chronic pain caused by inflammatory bowel disease

- Systemic lupus erythematosus (SLE): the most common type of lupus, an autoimmune disease

- Recurrent sickle cell disease crises

- Chronic ischemic heart disease

Not all patients with chronic pain have sensitization of the pain system, although most do. A rare example of chronic nociceptive pain without sensitization is arthritis of a joint, when the surgeon replaces that joint with a new artificial joint and the pain goes away completely.

Central Sensitization

Acute pain and chronic pain affect the pain system differently.

After an acute injury, the tissues heal. A fracture heals, a skin burn becomes a scar and a disk herniation is reabsorbed.

Chronic pain is more complex than acute pain. If pain persists after an injury, it is very likely not a sign that the injury is still there. It is a sign that the pain system has become sensitized.

When acute pain becomes chronic, we begin to see changes in the pain system. We've already talked a bit about nociplastic pain, which occurs when the pain system is sensitized. We refer to this change as *central sensitization.*

Central sensitization means that the spinal cord is modified to become more sensitive to pain. These changes, which occur as a response to persistent or ongoing acute pain, change the pain system so that it becomes dysfunctional.

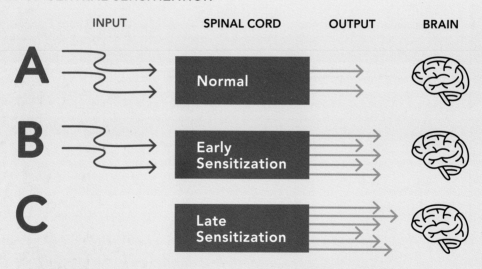

STAGES OF CENTRAL SENSITIZATION

INPUT   SPINAL CORD   OUTPUT   BRAIN

A — Normal

B — Early Sensitization

C — Late Sensitization

A: The pain is normal. The input and output are proportional. The brain receives information that is proportional to the intensity of injury.

B: The pain system is sensitized. The output is disproportional to the input. The brain receives information that there is a large damaged area and/or the damage is very severe.

C: Late stages of sensitization. There is no input. The injury is healed or the disease is treated. Yet the brain continues receiving information about a large area of severe damage.

Figure above adapted from Nijs (2011).

In fact, a person with chronic pain may not need nociception to feel pain. In other words, they don't need a sensor for the pain to start the process of activating the pain system. The whole pain system stays active without being stimulated. The pain system does not need a painful stimulus to continue being active.

Don't worry; I am not saying that your pain is not real. If you feel pain, then it is real. What is different is where the pain is originating. This is important, because our success in conquering pain is much higher if we start working with a person who is early in the transition from acute to chronic pain. It is easier to revert early central sensitization than it is to revert late central sensitization.

> **If you feel pain, then it is real.**

Sensitization is change that occurs in specific parts of the pain system. Peripheral sensitization occurs in the peripheral nerves and central sensitization occurs in the spinal cord.

Nociplastic pain is caused by sensitization and many other changes. Sensitization is just one of the changes. It is the one that has been most studied in the past 20 years. (Other changes that lead to nociplastic pain include altered cerebral pain processing, hormonal and immunological responses to pain.)

Thinking about pain can cause you to feel pain

The pain system has been sensitized by a previous pain (an acute pain), but now it does not need the acute pain anymore. It can activate itself.

This is the same mechanism as memory. You need to learn something first. But after you learn, you can remember things forever. The more you practice, the better you get at it.

The more a person thinks about pain, the stronger that memory of being in pain gets, and the stronger and more intensely they feel that pain. The synapses between the neurons get stronger and make it easy for the information to travel automatically.

Think about when you first learned to drive. You had to create synapses in your brain that connected the vision, hearing and touch sensations to the movements of the arms, legs, eyes and neck. In the beginning, you had to make a conscious effort to pay attention to all the information that was coming to your brain, use your judgment to make the wiser decisions and control the movement of your whole body. Now, after many years, you can drive automatically; you can even have a nice chat with the passenger at your side or listen to the radio. That is because the synapses that you made were reinforced. They became stronger and stronger, and you don't need to make any effort for the electrical impulses to travel from one side of your brain to the other and to the whole body.

When a person has pain for 10, 20, 30 years or more, their pain synapses are so strong that they feel pain even without the need to be conscious of it. It is an automatic reaction. They became experts.

The sooner you start deconstructing those synapses, the better. You want to do this before they become too strong.

Sensitization means we need to fix the alarm system

Sensitization can occur in the peripheral nerves and in the spinal cord. When there is sensitization of the pain system, we need to fix the alarm system. If the house's alarm system is malfunctioning, and there is no burglar, broken pipe or fire, then we need to call the alarm company, not the police, plumber or firefighter.

When a person understands the concept of sensitization, they don't ask me how to eliminate their pain. That would be like calling the firefighters to silence the alarm when the problem is a malfunctioning alarm system. Instead, they call the alarm company.

It is a waste of time and resources to call the firefighters, ambulance or police when the alarm system is malfunctioning. And the homeowner may even get a fine for calling emergency services frequently for false alarms.

The same principle applies to fixing nociplastic pain. Once your pain system has become sensitized, it is a waste of time to try fixing the area of the body that is hurting, because that is not where the problem is anymore. The problem has been transferred to the pain system. The important question is how to fix your pain system.

"The question that I want to hear from my patients is 'How can I fix my pain system?'"

Is My Pain All in My Head?

People with nociplastic pain usually have pain in more than one area of their body. They often have other symptoms of central sensitization and brain reorganization, which can include poor concentration, poor sleep, sensitivity to light, noise and smells, low mood, anxiety, irritability, itchiness and numbness.

They have tried all kinds of therapies and nothing works. They have been subjected to multiple investigations with radiological images, blood tests and even exploratory surgeries. And yet no one finds what is causing the pain.

People with nociplastic pain are the ones who are told "your pain is in your head," "there is nothing wrong with you," or "this pain is psychological."

Very few physicians are trained to diagnose nociplastic pain. (See the next chapter, *Getting a Diagnosis.*) What is most sad is that when the doctors don't know what it is, they prescribe multiple medications, perform injections and prescribe treatments that do not work for nociplastic pain, or could even be making it worse. For instance, they may prescribe opioids, which are known to worsen central sensitization, when there are much better ways to tackle nociplastic pain. (See *Step 6: Check Your Medicine Cabinet* for a discussion about using opioids for pain.)

> People with nociplastic pain are the ones who are told "your pain is in your head." Very few physicians are trained to diagnose nociplastic pain.

CONGENITAL INSENSITIVITY TO PAIN

There is a rare disease called congenital insensitivity to pain (CIP). Congenital means that the person is born with this disease. Individuals affected by CIP never feel pain. They do not have the ability to feel pain, so they lack awareness of dangerous situations and cannot protect themselves from injuries. They grow up with many wounds, bruises, fractures and burns. They bite their own tongues and don't feel pain. They don't avoid dangerous situations because they don't feel them as a threat. Fortunately, this is a very rare disease, because they usually die at an early age due to the multiple injuries they have received.

Therefore, having some pain is good. It protects us and prevents us from engaging in harmful experiences and situations. When a person feels pain, they tend to avoid that situation, or they try to be more careful or use safer methods the next time.

All pain is real

You may wonder, if you are told that your pain is all in your head, if your pain is actually real. *Pain from central sensitization*, which is created in the brain without painful stimulation, is very real and very painful. Sometimes, just moving the body part or rubbing the skin with a cotton ball will trigger pain.

Remember, your brain does not need a painful stimulus to feel pain. It is capable of activating itself without a nociceptive (painful) stimulus. All it needs is to be convinced that there is a danger. Then, in an attempt to preserve your life, your brain will trigger a cascade of brain waves that will be interpreted as pain.

I call this a painful illusion. Something similar happens with optical illusions and auditory illusions. The eye can see one image, but the brain will interpret it as a different thing. Or the ears will hear a sound but the brain will interpret it as a different sound.

"All pain is real."

THERE IS NOTHING WRONG

When you look at an optical illusion and see something that is not there, it does not mean there is something wrong with your eyes; it is just your mind misinterpreting a visual sensation. In the case of nociplastic pain, there is nothing wrong with the area where you are feeling pain. It is just a sensory illusion. The brain is trying to tell you there is danger, but there is nothing to be fixed. You need to understand and believe that.

PAIN IS REAL, BUT IN THE CASE OF NOCIPLASTIC PAIN, YOUR BRAIN IS LYING TO YOU.

Pain is real and it is annoying, constant, tiring and depressing. Well, that is what your brain is telling you and in the case of nociplastic pain, that is a lie. Your brain is lying to you.

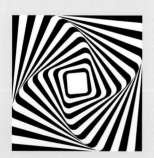

Look at this picture. Your brain is probably telling you that these lines are curved.

Your brain is lying to you.

These lines are not curved. They come from perfect squares.

If you don't believe this, turn to page 38.

In 1995, there was a report in the BMJ medical journal *Minerva* of a 29-year-old construction worker who was rushed to the emergency department after having jumped down onto a 6-inch (15 cm) nail. The nail went all the way through his boot, transfixing him to the spot, and was visible on the top of the boot.

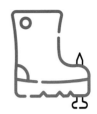

Any small movement caused terrible pain, so they had to give him fentanyl and midazolam to sedate him to pull the nail from below. When the boot was removed, they noticed that the skin was intact and that the nail had passed between his toes.

Who will say that his pain was not real? It was real, but it did not need painful stimulation to start the process. All it needed was the pain centers in the brain to become activated.

This is actually good news, because if the pain system can be activated just by believing there is a threat, it can also be deactivated by believing that the threat is removed.

In the next chapter, *Getting a Diagnosis,* we will see how doctors diagnose the type of pain you have. If you are diagnosed with nociplastic pain, you should be happy right now. You know why? Because in the same way that the pain system can malfunction and generate pain sensations, it can also be retrained to stop all these pain sensations. I've seen that many times. You need to believe, and then you will see.

> **If your doctor diagnoses you with *nociplastic pain,* that is good news. It means your pain can be eliminated by retraining your pain system.**

TECHNICAL TERMS

NOCICEPTIVE PAIN: Activated by nociceptors, or pain sensors, in our skin and other organs
NEUROPATHIC PAIN: Activated by injury or disease to our peripheral or central nerve system
NOCIPLASTIC PAIN: Originates from a malfunction of our pain system

Fixing Your Alarm System

When you have nociplastic pain, your brain is trying to protect you from danger. Yet nociplastic pain does not protect you from anything. It is a false alarm. It is the alarm that is malfunctioning.

The good news is, because your brain has the ability to create these false alarms, your brain also has the ability to erase them. The sooner you start, the better the results. Early phases of central sensitization are easier to revert than late phases.

Fixing the alarm system of the body, or the pain system, is very rewarding. It is what gives me most joy in my profession.

When someone asks me "Dr. Furlan, why did you choose to be a pain doctor? It must be terrible hearing people complaining of their pains if you can't cure them!" My response is this: "Even if I can't cure the pain that a person has, I can help to improve the person who has pain."

I have seen hundreds, if not thousands of people conquering their chronic pain mountain. Each person has a different story. Each mountain is different.

I am here to help them as they climb. Once they are at the top, they discharge me. They don't need to come to our pain clinic anymore. Or they come once a year just to tell me their progress and latest adventures.

> You should not let pain dictate what you do or not do. Yes, that is easier said than done. But it is possible.

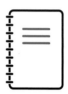

What will the top of the mountain look like for you?

What kind of pain do you think you have?

Let's do an exercise. You are not supposed to diagnose your own type of pain. You need a doctor to tell you what kind of pain you have. Get your journal and answer these questions:

1. What did the doctors tell you is your pain type? Nociceptive, neuropathic or nociplastic?

2. How many different diagnoses have you been given for your pain? Compare with the list on page 31.

3. How many pills have you taken in your whole life for this pain? How many surgeries? How many injections?

This book is about giving you knowledge and tools that you can use to discuss your pain with your doctor.

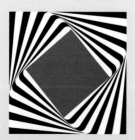

Look at this image compared to the image on page 36. You can see here that the lines are actually straight in the previous optical illusion.

CONCLUSION

The information I have shared in this chapter is based on the latest discoveries in pain neuroscience. Although not an exhaustive list, it includes some of the amazing science of how pain works in our body. Knowing these concepts makes a good foundation for conquering your pain.

KEY POINTS TO REMEMBER

- We have a pain system installed in our bodies. Its function is to protect us from injuries and diseases by alerting our mind that there is some danger that needs to be removed.
- Like an alarm system in a house, the pain system can malfunction. This process is called sensitization.
- Sensitization makes the brain more sensitive to pain; it increases the pain volume and intensifies other sensations, including touch, noise and body movements. Sensitization can also generate the perception of pain in the brain even when there is no danger to the body.
- There are three kinds of pain: nociceptive, neuropathic and nociplastic. When the pain system is malfunctioning, we call this nociplastic pain.
- All pain is real.
- The amount of pain we feel is not a good measure of how much injury or disease is affecting our body
- It is possible to fix the pain system. The first step is to understand and accept the type of pain you have.

LOOKING AHEAD

In the next chapter, *Getting a Diagnosis,* we'll visit a typical pain clinic and see what is involved in getting a diagnosis.

- You will learn how you can explain your pain to your doctor.
- You will understand what questions your doctor needs to ask you and the physical examination they need to do to diagnose if your pain is nociceptive, neuropathic, nociplastic or mixed.

Getting a Diagnosis

Before taking on the mountain, the aspiring mountaineer has to have a physical check-up, pass a fitness test and get the appropriate training. They do this by joining a club, a team or a group of professional individuals who have the expertise and experience to guide them on their journey.

In this chapter, we will talk about the many experts who can help you to conquer your chronic pain. Whether you go to a pain doctor or a pain clinic, they will usually ask you a lot of questions about your pain, your life and your goals. We will also talk about how doctors diagnose the various types of pain, and we will introduce you to the "toolbox" of strategies to conquer your pain.

Pain Doctors

The journey to becoming a pain specialist can include up to 15 years of study and practice:

- Undergraduate university program (three to four years)
- Medical school (four years)
- Residency (two years for family medicine, or four to five years for other specialties)
- Pain fellowship or pain residency (two years)

Doctors who specialize in pain come from various medical fields, including physical medicine and rehabilitation, anesthesia, psychiatry, neurology, rheumatology, orthopedic surgery, general internal medicine, family medicine and pediatrics.

Pain doctors can work in private practice or at a hospital. They can be independent of a university or affiliated with a medical school. They can work by themselves, in a pain team or pain clinic. Scientific studies have demonstrated that multidisciplinary pain teams achieve better results with chronic pain than those with only a single discipline. This makes sense, as we are treating the whole person and not just the pain.

Multidisciplinary means that there are experts in various disciplines in the clinic. These can include doctors of various specialties, nurses, pharmacists, psychologists, physical and occupational therapists, social workers, dietitians and more.

The Visit to a Pain Clinic

The first time you are seen at a pain clinic, you may see only one professional or many simultaneously. It depends on the clinic's structure. The first professional you see may be a physician, a nurse, a nurse practitioner or another healthcare professional such as physiotherapist, psychologist or social worker.

The initial visit may feel overwhelming, as you will be providing a lot of information. You may be asked to complete a number of questionnaires and interviews with different professionals.

What the doctor will ask you

The information patients are asked for at the initial assessment usually includes:

DEMOGRAPHICS
- **AGE:** Some diseases affect age groups differently. For example, osteoarthritis is more common in older people, while rheumatoid arthritis usually starts at an earlier age.
- **SEX:** There are diseases that affect men and women differently. Gout affects more men than women, and fibromyalgia affects more women.
- **MARITAL STATUS AND FAMILY MEMBERS:** It is good to know if the you have a spouse or family that could be involved in the management of your chronic pain.
- **EMPLOYMENT STATUS:** The healthcare team will ask you about your ability to stay at work or return to work.

- **JOB TITLE:** It is also important to get information about what you do at work and their work environment, for example, if it involves heavy lifting, repetitive movements, awkward positions, hazardous situations or toxic substances.

YOUR GOALS

Your pain team will ask you what you hope to get out of this clinic or program. What are your expectations? We work with patients to develop specific goals and not just general goals such as "improve my pain." (We discuss SMARTer goals in *Step 8: Focus on Your Goals.*)

SPECIFIC QUESTIONNAIRES

You may also be asked to complete questionnaires that help to assess your mood, anxiety, beliefs and fears, and how ready you are to embark on significant changes in your pain management.

CHARACTERISTICS OF YOUR PAIN

A body pain diagram

You will be given a body pain diagram and asked to paint, color or shade all areas where you experience pain.

For example:

❶ This pain drawing suggests that the pain is all localized in the joints: left and right shoulders, hands, hips, knees and ankles. This might indicate there is some sort of inflammatory arthritis or osteoarthritis.

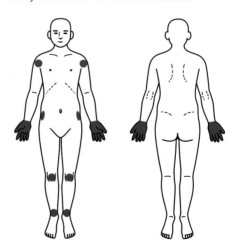

2 This pain drawing suggests that there is central sensitization (nociplastic pain), as in the case of fibromyalgia.

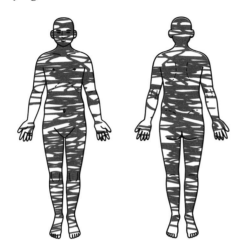

The body pain diagram is one of the most valuable tools that we have to make the diagnosis of chronic pain.

A description of your pain

They will ask you to describe your pain. Specifically, you will be asked about the onset of pain, characteristics, radiation (where it starts and where else you feel it), associated symptoms, timing, what makes it feel better (or worse) and the severity.

What does the pain feel like? Can you describe how you feel this pain? Here are some examples: hot, burning, electrical shocks, ice-cold, tiring, heavy, diffuse, throbbing, numbing.

How long have you had this pain? Is it constant or intermittent? Is there a time of the day when the pain is worse? Pain that is worse when you wake up suggests inflammatory arthritis. Pain that is worse after a full day of work suggests muscle strain and myofascial trigger points.

What makes it worse and better? Does movement make it worse or better? How about anxiety, frustration and sadness? Do you take painkillers? How much is the pain improved with painkillers? Does it get better with heat or ice? If the pain gets better with ice, it is likely inflammation; but if it gets worse with ice, then it is likely neuropathic. If the pain gets better with NSAIDs, then it suggests inflammation; if it gets better with antidepressants and anticonvulsants, it suggests neuropathic pain. If the pain goes away completely when you are meditating, that suggests nociplastic pain.

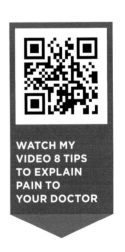

WATCH MY VIDEO 8 TIPS TO EXPLAIN PAIN TO YOUR DOCTOR

SOCRATES

I use the SOCRATES method to get the information I need about pain.

S is the site. Where does it hurt?

O is the onset. What were you doing when the pain started?

C is for characteristics. What does the pain feel like?

R is for radiation. Does it go anywhere else?

A is for associated symptoms and ameliorating factors

T is for time. When did it start? When do you feel it most?

E is for exacerbating. What makes it worse or better?

S is for severity or pain intensity.

MEASURING PAIN

We ask patients to assign a number to how much pain they are feeling, but that question can be hard to answer and the answer can be difficult to interpret.

We usually ask for a number from 0 to 10. If they say 8, 9 or 10, we tend to be worried that the patient is suffering a lot. Yet this number is a composite of a lot of information.

The number may reflect the pain sensation itself, but it can be inflated by other concerns and worries. Such issues include fear of what might be causing the pain, worry about the future, doubt that the diagnosis is correct, worry about physical disability or disfiguration, uncertainty about the competence of the physician, lack of support from a family member or coworkers, financial consequences, perception of self-worth and self-esteem, social role and status, and ability to maintain a job, finish school, get married, have children or take a vacation.

Even if you find it hard to assign a number to your pain, this part of the consult is important. First, we need to know if there is ever a time that your pain is zero. If there is a chance that your pain can get to zero, then it is easier to come up with a treatment plan. Also, we need to compare your pain severity scores before and after you try any treatments.

For more about measuring pain, and how to speak with your doctor about your pain, see page 163 in *Step 5: Get Help from Others*. See also pages 192–193.

PAIN MEDICATIONS

The pain doctor needs to know all the medications that you are currently taking as well as those you have tried in the past. This includes prescription, over-the-counter, vitamins, supplements and natural medicine, including any others besides the ones for pain.

You will be asked to provide the following information:

- Medication name
- Dose and number taken daily
- How long you have been taking it
- How well it works (a lot, a little, not at all)
- If you have any adverse reaction to this medication

OTHER TREATMENTS

You may be asked what treatments you have tried for this pain condition and to rate them as not tried, very helpful, a little helpful or not helpful. Possibilities include massage, chiropractic, acupuncture, physiotherapy, exercises, mental health counseling, mindfulness, meditation, other mind-body therapies, heat, cold and other therapies.

HEALTH HISTORY

We also need to get a general sense of your overall health, habits, family and your personal history:

- Substance use (nicotine, alcohol, recreational drugs)
- Family history (hereditary disorders, health issues, etc.)
- Allergies (to medications, food, substances, environmental substances, etc.)
- Past medical history and surgeries, even going back to your childhood

HOW DO DOCTORS DIAGNOSE CHRONIC PAIN?
With the information from your history, physical exam and questionnaires, the physician usually has enough details to make a diagnosis of your pain condition. Rarely do we need to order tests to make a diagnosis.

With the information provided above, your doctor will have an idea of what the pain diagnosis is. They will have some hypotheses. The next step is to test these hypotheses by doing a thorough physical examination.

The physical exam follows a structured sequence of tests and observations.

OBSERVATION

The doctor will observe and document your appearance, mood and gait (the way you walk and stand), plus any deformity or postural differences, as well as your cooperation with the exam. You may be too tired, depressed and frustrated that day, in which case the doctor may conclude that a physical exam will not be optimal and should be repeated another time. The doctor will also note any assistive devices, such as crutches, wheelchair or a walker, that you use.

VITAL SIGNS

The doctor or nurse will check your vital signs, including blood pressure, heart rate, oximetry and respiratory rate.

MUSCULOSKELETAL EXAMINATION

If your pain involves muscles, tendons and bones, the physician will do special tests for each body part. They will look for any redness, deformity, swelling or change in temperature and range of motion. They will feel around the affected body area, and perform specific checks to test the stability of the joints, how movement is impaired and how the symptoms can be reproduced.

NEUROLOGICAL EXAM

A neurological exam is done when the physician needs to test your brain, spinal cord or peripheral nerve functions. The doctor will observe tremors, muscle atrophies, deformities, skin marks, nails, hair, sweating and temperature.

The exam involves mainly two areas: the motor system and the sensory system.

The motor system includes all functions controlled by the brain, such as eyes movement, tongue, muscles, balance and gait.

The sensory system includes all information that is brought to the brain. Testing the sensory system may include a light touch, pin prick, vibration, heat, cold or deep pressure. The doctor will be looking for abnormalities of the sensory system, such as numbness or hypersensitivity to touch.

Diagnostic tests, laboratory and imaging studies

The doctor may order diagnostic tests, laboratory or imaging studies to confirm what they suspect from a patient's history and physical exam.

For example, a patient's pain diagram suggests a disk herniation on the neck, with pain mainly going to the shoulder and arm. The physical examination shows that certain muscles on the right side are weaker, and that the triceps reflex, which is a related to those muscles, is absent. That suggests the patient has a specific cervical radiculopathy (a pinched nerve at the C7 level) that is causing the pain in the arm.

The doctor may order a nerve conduction study (NCS) with electromyography (EMG) on the right arm to confirm the diagnosis and to document the nerve fibers that are affected by the disk herniation. A CT scan or a magnetic resonance image (MRI) of the cervical spine may be ordered to see if the radiculopathy is caused by a compression of the nerve, which most commonly is a disk herniation. But there are other causes of radiculopathy that are not related to the disks, for example, a varicela zoster infection.

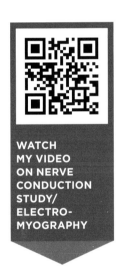

WATCH MY VIDEO ON NERVE CONDUCTION STUDY/ ELECTRO-MYOGRAPHY

They may also order blood tests to rule out other conditions like lupus, rheumatoid arthritis, thyroid problems, vitamin B_{12} deficiency, anemia, kidney or liver diseases.

AN OBSESSION WITH MRIS AND OTHER IMAGING STUDIES

There seems to be an obsession with MRIs and other imaging studies these days. Too many people rely on them, thinking they will provide the answers to "where the problem is coming from." This attitude is perpetuated by doctors who do not know how to properly examine a patient with chronic pain, and patients who demand their doctors order more and more exams to find where the pain is coming from.

Remember, nociplastic pain does not show up on regular brain CT scans or MR imaging. The only way to diagnose it is by excluding nociceptive or neuropathic pain, and by detecting a pattern of symptoms and physical examination signs that are very typical.

This quest to find an image that shows where the pain is coming from leads to an enormous number of useless exams and wasted time and money. It is not rare to see patients who have repeated the same exams over and over for many years.

I have had many patients come to see me bringing dozens of MRIs and other image studies along with them. None of these image studies was correlated to the findings from their history and physical examination.

So, why do so many doctors order an MRI? The answer is simple. It takes 30 to 60 minutes to take a good history and perform a complete physical examination. And it takes only five minutes to order an MRI. Most doctors don't have the time or they don't even know where to start.

But is there a problem with replacing the person's history and physical with an MRI? Yes, there is a huge problem. The MRI will always show something is wrong. The MR images are so sensitive that they can show many abnormalities that do not have any clinical importance.

The results of imaging studies are only relevant if they are directly related to the patient's symptoms and they match exactly what the physical examination demonstrated.

THE ONLY TIME IN YOUR LIFE THAT YOU WILL HAVE A NORMAL MRI IS WHEN YOU ARE A NEWBORN BABY

There is no single person in this world who will have a completely normal MRI of their body. Okay, that is a slight exaggeration. Maybe one percent of people — and those are newborn babies only — would have normal MRIs.

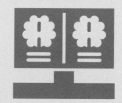

"Remember, nociplastic pain does not show up on regular brain CT scans or MR imaging."

ABNORMALITIES DON'T NECESSARILY MEAN PAIN

When we do spine MRIs of people without back pain, a great proportion of them will have some abnormality. The older you are, the higher the chances of finding "serious" abnormalities such as disk herniation and spinal stenosis.

If we do X-rays of the knees, hips, shoulders, neck and lumbar spine of people without pain, the majority of them will have some abnormality. The older you get, the higher the chances of finding abnormalities such as osteoarthritis, osteophytes, bone erosion and cysts.

But why did all these people with abnormalities not have any pain? The answer is simple. Pain is not a measure of how much injury there is in a body part. Pain intensity is not proportional to the size or degree of an injury or illness. A person may have a very tiny injury or no injury, and feel a lot of pain. (Recall the story of the construction worker who had excruciating pain without the nail actually entering his skin, on page 37 of this book.) On the other hand, a person may have a very serious injury or illness and have no pain at all.

In a 2015 study (Brinjikii et al.), more than 3,000 random people without back pain were subjected to MRIs of the lumbar spine. Many of them were found to have disk degeneration, disk bulge and disk protrusion. Older individuals had more of these problems than younger individuals, yet they too were asymptomatic and were not even aware of these problems. (See the figure below, based on the study results.)

> **Pain is not a measure of how much injury there is in a body part. Pain intensity is not proportional to the size or degree of an injury or illness.**

PROPORTION OF ABNORMAL MRIS AMONG PEOPLE WHO ARE ASYMPTOMATIC AND DO NOT HAVE ANY BACK PAIN SYMPTOMS

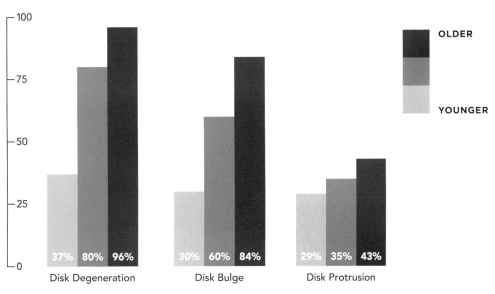

OLDER

YOUNGER

	Disk Degeneration	Disk Bulge	Disk Protrusion
Younger	37%	30%	29%
Middle	80%	60%	35%
Older	96%	84%	43%

TERRY AND THE SURGEON WHO PLANTED THE SEEDS OF PAIN

Terry was very athletic and going to the gym many times a week, yet had many episodes of low back pain every year. Still, her pain was under control.

Then one day she saw an orthopedic surgeon, and this doctor told her she had terrible arthritis in her spine and that it would get worse and worse. She heard from this doctor that there was no cure for arthritis of the spine and that she would have to learn how to live with this problem.

Well, her back pain started getting worse, she stopped going to the gym, withdrew from social activities, developed depression and now was on multiple medications for chronic pain. And the pain was constant and very intense, even though she was taking multiple painkillers every day.

That orthopedic doctor planted a seed in her head, that she would get worse. She believed what the doctor said and she watered that seed every day. It grew and became a very large tree.

Now, my job was to help her cut down that tree. I told her: "You have to unlearn what the orthopedic doctor told you." Eventually she was able to stop taking all painkillers, went back to the gym and her depression vanished.

In my pain clinic, I have had to spend many hours undoing what other physicians have told my patients.

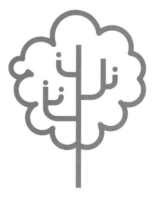

Mark and Mike

Mark is a 30-year-old man who has had cerebral palsy since birth. His knees, hips and feet have severe deformities. He has had multiple surgeries to correct the shortened tendons. The X-rays and MRIs of his joints show very severe osteoarthritis. His shoulders have multiple areas of compression of tendons and bone abnormalities because he uses a walker.

Mike is a 26-year-old man who works 12 hours a day as an office assistant. His manager is very demanding and his coworkers are lazy. He is the only one in the office who knows how to do the job well, so his boss keeps giving him more and more work, while the other staff are always chatting in the kitchen about the latest TV show. He doesn't have time to watch TV, as he is always exhausted. His X-rays and MRIs of the neck do not show any severe abnormality.

Who has chronic pain? Mark or Mike?

If you see Mark's X-rays and MRIs, you will think he is in constant, terrible, excruciating pain 24 hours a day. But it is quite the opposite. Mark does not have any pain. Mike has constant pain in his upper neck and shoulders and chronic migraines.

Why Some People Have Chronic Pain and Others Don't

There are many factors that are associated with a predisposition to chronic pain. Some factors have been studied in excellent research studies, but others are still being investigated by scientists around the world. There is not a single factor but many factors that may lead to chronic pain, especially nociplastic pain. They are described in the table on the following page.

Adverse childhood experiences

Having adverse childhood experiences (ACEs) predisposes a person not only to chronic pain and fibromyalgia, but also to a lot of other health conditions. The more adverse childhood experiences a child has when growing up, the greater the chances of them having a health issue, including emotional difficulties in adult life (Felitti, Anda and Nordenberg, 1998). And adverse childhood experiences are very common. About 6 to 7 percent of the general population in the world will have at least one factor.

FACTORS INVOLVED IN THE TRANSITION
FROM ACUTE TO CHRONIC PAIN

BIOLOGICAL FACTORS	Injury or disease	Extent of the injury Condition of tissues or organs affected
	Body structures	Posture Muscle imbalances or weakness Congenital diseases
	Ability to heal	Nutrition Immune system Ongoing diseases: for example, diabetes, hypothyroidism Sleep quality Cardiovascular fitness Normal body mass index (BMI) Toxins: alcohol, smoke, caffeine, drugs
PSYCHOLOGICAL FACTORS	Mood	Depression, anxiety
	Personality traits	Catastrophization, perfectionism and people pleasing
	Trauma	Adverse childhood experiences (ACEs) Post-traumatic stress disorders (PTSDs)
SOCIAL FACTORS	Community	Social isolation, access to recreation
	Job	Job demands, supportive coworkers and managers Job control, work-life balance, perceived injustices
ENVIRONMENTAL FACTORS	Pollution	Air pollution, noise, unclean water and sanitation
	Green spaces	Nature, open spaces, public spaces
HEALTHCARE	Access	Preventive medicine, immunizations, screenings, mental health services
	Rehabilitation	Physiotherapy for acute injuries
	Surgery	Anesthesia, post-operatory pain management

The brain develops during childhood until maturity around the age of 18. This development can be affected by childhood trauma.

To learn about trauma-informed care for people with chronic pain, see page [xx] in *Step 2: Control Your Emotions.*

- The ***prefrontal cortex***, which is the thinking center in the front of the brain, will be underactivated and this may be reflected in difficulties concentrating and learning.
- The ***anterior cingulate cortex***, which is responsible for the emotional regulation, will also become underdeveloped, meaning that the person will have difficulties managing emotions in adult life.
- The ***amygdala***, the center for fear, will become overactivated, meaning that the person will have difficulty feeling safe, calming down and sleeping.

AREAS OF THE BRAIN AFFECTED BY ADVERSE CHILDHOOD EXPERIENCES

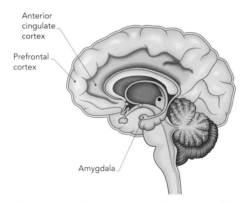

Anterior cingulate cortex

Prefrontal cortex

Amygdala

The scientific research community has named 10 types of adverse childhood experiences. They are categorized into three main categories: abuse, neglect and household dysfunction.

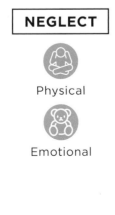

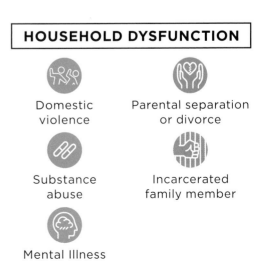

ABUSE	NEGLECT	HOUSEHOLD DYSFUNCTION	
Physical	Physical	Domestic violence	Parental separation or divorce
Emotional	Emotional	Substance abuse	Incarcerated family member
Sexual		Mental Illness	

How Do Doctors Diagnose the Type of Pain?

How do doctors diagnose what type of pain you have?

The answer lies in a good medical evaluation. A clinician trained in pain management will be able to assess a patient with chronic pain and determine if there is sensitization or not. The table below describes some of the things a clinician will look for.

THREE KINDS OF PAIN

	NOCICEPTIVE	NEUROPATHIC	NOCIPLASTIC
Area	Localized to a specific part of the body	Restricted to the area related to the peripheral or central nervous system lesion	Spread to many areas; does not confine to a neurological distribution
Characteristics	Aching, sore, inflamed, sharp, colic, spasms, pressure	Burning, pins and needles, electrical shocks, numbness, throbbing	Diffuse, heavy, tingling, tiring, pressure, numbing
Physical signs	Redness, swelling, hot, deformity. Physical exam positive and consistent for specific tests and maneuvers	Abnormal sensations that follow the distribution of the innervated area. Muscle atrophy or weakness; abnormal reflexes; other neurological signs	Abnormal sensations do not follow a pattern of innervation. Otherwise, a normal neurological exam
Mental status	Some anxiety related to pain. May affect sleep quality	Mild, moderate or severe effects on psychological status	Mild to severe effects on mental status. Fatigue, poor concentration, mental fog, hopeless and helpless
Number of previous diagnostic tests and visits to physicians	Few	Moderate	Many diagnostic tests with negative results. Many visits to various specialists

	NOCICEPTIVE	NEUROPATHIC	NOCIPLASTIC
Previous treatments attempted to alleviate this pain	Few, with good response	Moderate to many, with good response	Many failed attempts. A lot of time and money spent trying to figure out a cure
Time to reach a stable treatment	Days, weeks or a few months	Weeks to months	Many years to decades
Sleep disturbance	Minimal	Moderate	Severe
Ability to function	Minimally or moderately impaired	Minimally or moderately impaired	Moderately to severely impaired
Response to opioids	Improves	Improves	Gets worse; opioids increase central sensitization
Response to acetaminophen and NSAIDs	Big improvement	A little improvement	No improvement
Response to antidepressants and anticonvulsants	A little improvement	Big improvement	A little improvement
Response to exercises	Big improvement	A little improvement	Big improvement, but have to start low and go slow
Response to mind-body therapies	Some improvement	Some improvement	Big improvement
Response to manual therapies	Some improvement	No improvement. May get worse if the person has allodynia (pain when touching the skin)	No improvement
Response to modalities (heat, cold, TENS)	Big improvement	A little improvement. May get worse with cold	No improvement
Response to injections and nerve blocks	Big improvement	Big improvement	Gets worse; painful injections provoke more central sensitization
Response to surgery	Big improvement if the cause can be well identified	Improvement if the cause is a nerve compression	Gets worse; painful surgeries provoke more central sensitization

What Happens Next?

The pain clinic team will generate a report about your diagnosis(es) and treatment plan.

If the clinician reports on your pain using terms like "sensitization of the pain system," or "nociplastic pain" or "fibromyalgia," that means that your alarm system is showing some signs of malfunctioning and sensitization.

If you have a family doctor, nurse practitioner or other primary care clinician, they will likely receive a copy of this report. They will help you to find resources close to your home and follow your progress. You may need to return to the pain clinic for more appointments, investigations, more questionnaires or educational group sessions.

How much pain relief can you expect?

When I ask my many patients with chronic pain how much pain relief they want, I get two types of response:

I want this pain 100 percent eliminated OR **I want my life back as before**

I have never met a patient who did not want their pain eliminated. That is what I want, too. There is nothing wrong with wanting that, but this wish often comes with three huge problems.

1. *Patients want me to cure their pain.* They want me to give them a magic pill, an injection, an exercise, something that will make their pain go away. If their expectations are not met, they get frustrated and keep going from doctor to doctor with the same expectations.

2. *There are some kinds of pain that will be part of my patient's lives permanently.* And then the question is, can they still live a better life today? They may not want to hear this, but their life will not return to what it was before. They will need to reframe their life as is now.

3. *They are so occupied in finding a cure that they neglect living their lives during the journey.* For them, the destination is what matters, not the trip. It is like the kid in the car who keeps asking "Are we there yet?" for hours instead of watching movies, playing games or napping.

By the time most people get to me, a chronic pain specialist, they have already developed a disease of the pain system. Because of central sensitization, their pain system has been modified by pain. It is still possible to revert it, but the sooner we start, the better the results. We will talk more about that in the next chapter, *Step 1: Retrain Your Pain System*.

What if I have all three kinds of pain?

I have seen many patients who have two or all three types of pain. For example, low back pain can be a mix of nociceptive (trigger points in the muscles), neuropathic (compression of a nerve root exiting the spinal cord) and nociplastic pain (resulting from sensitization).

Another example is cancer-related pain. Nowadays many more people are surviving cancer, or living many years with cancer therapies. However, they are constantly being exposed to acute pain, either by the cancer growth itself, or the surgeries, chemotherapy or radiotherapy treatments. Most of these treatments also cause injuries to peripheral nerves, leading to neuropathic pain. But cancer patients are always hypervigilant with pain. They are terrified of any pain sensation, because that can be linked to tumor growth or metastases. Almost all cancer patients develop sensitization of the pain system and fear of pain.

Other examples of mixed types of pain may include arthritis, sickle cell diseases, hypermobility, migraine, irritable bowel syndrome, TMJ dysfunction and back pain.

WHICH TYPE OF PAIN IS EASIER TO ELIMINATE: NOCICEPTIVE, NEUROPATHIC OR NOCIPLASTIC?

The strategies differ, but all three kinds of pain can be eliminated completely. We use many tools to tackle pain from different perspectives.

There are a few treatments that help with more than one type of pain, for example, mind-body and movement interventions. For this reason, you will read a lot in this book about the benefits of movement and mind-body exercises.

People with chronic pain from mixed types are very satisfied when we reduce sensitization, as then it becomes much easier to identify and treat nociceptive and neuropathic pain. Why? It is easier to detect nociceptive or neuropathic pain when there is no amplification from sensitization.

> Once we eliminate sensitization, it becomes much easier to treat nociceptive and neuropathic pain. Why? It is much easier to detect and eliminate nociceptive and neuropathic pain when there is no amplification from sensitization.

Patients tell me that they still have the nociceptive or neuropathic pain, but now, their pain is less than before. They say that it doesn't interfere with their lives and it doesn't scare them anymore. They understand their own pain system, can manage their chronic pain and return to a state where they enjoy life.

And I have had patients with purely nociplastic pain. Once they conquer it, they are 100 percent pain free. But still they need to continue practicing the strategies they learned to prevent the pain from coming back.

 ## Meet Your Toolbox: Seven Types of Tools to Treat Pain

Let me introduce you to the toolbox! Throughout this book we will be referring to the tools inside it. I call these seven types of tools the 5M IS. This is a preview of *Step 7: Make Room in Your Toolbox.*

SEVEN TYPES OF TOOLS TO TREAT PAIN: 5M IS

M	**MIND-BODY THERAPIES:** cognitive behavioral therapy (CBT), acceptance and commitment therapy (ACT), mindfulness, meditation, prayer, hypnosis, biofeedback, graded motor imagery, mirror therapy, body scan, etc.
M	**MOVEMENT:** any kind of physical activity you enjoy: walking, dancing, swimming, biking, aerobics, cardio, strengthening with weights, stretching, relaxation, balance, yoga, tai chi, etc.
M	**MODALITIES:** application of heat, cold, electrotherapy, transcutaneous electrical nerve stimulation (TENS), taping, splints, braces, orthotics, ergonomic chair, pillows, mattress, acupuncture, etc.
M	**MANUAL THERAPIES:** massage, mobilization, manipulations, etc.
M	**MEDICATIONS:** analgesics, opioids, anti-inflammatories, muscle relaxants, antidepressants, anticonvulsants, cannabinoids, lidocaine, ketamine, steroids, etc.
I	**INTERVENTIONAL PAIN MANAGEMENT:** injections and nerve blocks, applied by trained medical professionals
S	**SURGICAL PROCEDURES:** joint replacements, nerve ablations, tendon repairs, spinal cord stimulators or deep brain stimulators

CONCLUSION

In the previous chapter, we learned the difference between chronic and acute pain, we explored the pain system and how it works like an alarm system, and I introduced you to the three kinds of pain and sensitization. In this chapter we reviewed what to expect at a pain clinic and how a doctor diagnoses chronic pain and determines what kind of pain you have. I also gave you a preview of our toolbox.

KEY POINTS TO REMEMBER

- Chronic pain may be too complex for a primary care provider. If possible, get a consult with a pain specialist in a multidisciplinary pain clinic.
- The pain clinic may need to do investigations, tests and questionnaires to determine the most likely diagnosis of your pain and to suggest a treatment plan.
- Most treatment plans can be followed by your primary care provider with resources close to your home.
- When you see your pain clinic team, ask questions and get as much education you can about your condition.

LOOKING AHEAD

Next, we are going to talk about the first step in your journey: how we can retrain the pain system, reduce central sensitization and treat nociplastic pain.

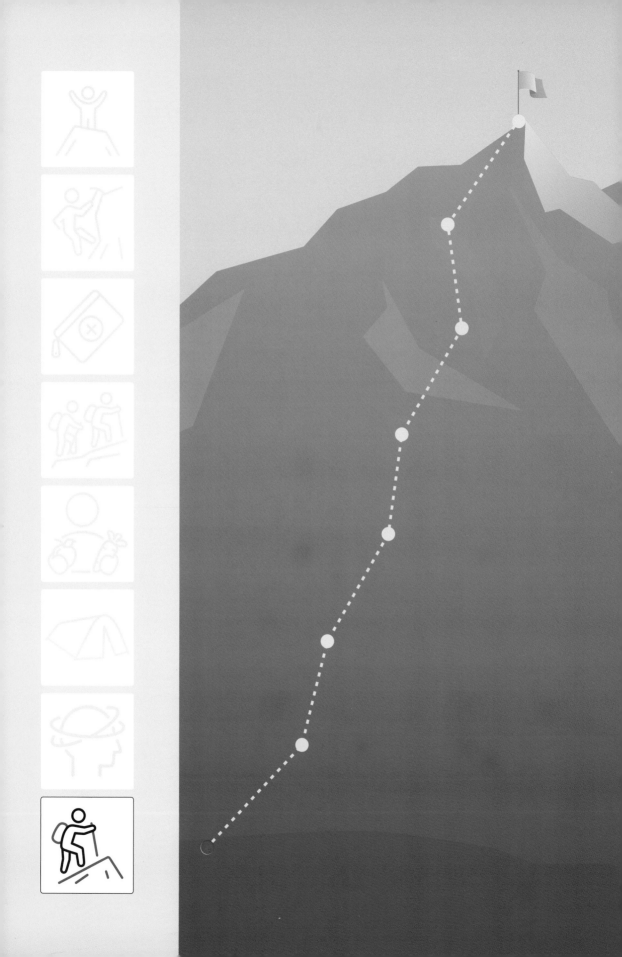

Retrain Your Pain System

Don't start the book here, with this chapter.

You will not understand what I mean by brain retraining if you skipped the previous chapters. You must understand the concept of **primary and secondary chronic pain.** Also, you need to be familiar with terms explained in earlier chapters, such as **nociceptive, neuropathic and nociplastic pain and sensitization** before you start reading this chapter.

The mountaineer cannot move to the next step if they don't understand that there is a mountain to be conquered. They may see the mountain but not believe they can climb it. Or they may see the mountain, believe they can climb it but not take the necessary steps to start climbing it. Climbing a mountain requires planning, studying, preparation and willingness. Not climbing the mountain means they will stay where they are and never see the top of the mountain or what lies on the other side.

In this chapter, we look at how to retrain your pain system to lessen or eliminate your pain. We begin by reviewing the concept of pain and kinds of pain, with a focus on nociplastic pain and the changes it makes in your brain. We learn how reducing nociplastic pain can help you control other kinds of pain. Then we look at the four stages of change, and your readiness to make changes. Then we get into the practical, proven steps you can take to use the mind-body connection to retrain your pain system and relieve your pain.

Nociplastic Pain: When Chronic Pain is the Disease Itself

In *What is Pain?* we saw that when pain is signaling that there is an injury or disease, then the pain is secondary. Nociceptive and neuropathic pain are both secondary pain.

When the injury or disease has healed and the person continues to feel pain, this is because the pain system has become sensitized. Then the pain is primary. Nociplastic pain is the mechanism for this primary chronic pain.

Primary chronic pain is a condition in which pain is the disease itself.

Nociplastic pain is the mechanism of primary chronic pain.

Central sensitization is one of the changes in the pain system that leads to nociplastic pain, probably the most important, and it is easier to revert when identified in the earlier stages.

In the previous chapters we learned about primary pain, and the technical term nociplastic pain. It is caused by sensitization of the pain system.

Do you have this type of pain? If you are not certain, ask your doctor to confirm your diagnosis. Many people with chronic pain have had their doctors tell them that there is nothing wrong with their body, that the pain is coming from their head. This is not an insult; it means that the doctor is telling them that their pain is nociplastic.

Remember, all pain is real, but in the case of nociplastic pain, your brain is trying to protect you by creating these painful sensations.

Often, a person with nociplastic pain will try multiple treatments, see many specialists and yet find that still nothing works. They may get different diagnoses from different clinicians. For some, it seems their pain is spreading to many parts of their body. In addition, they feel depressed, and are fatigued during the day and can't sleep at night. Does that sound familiar to you? These are often signs of central sensitization. The pain system has become sensitized.

Eliminating nociplastic pain can help you control the pain

Almost every patient with chronic pain has some component of nociplastic pain, especially if they have had pain for many years. They may have other kinds of pain as well. For example, a person with painful diabetic neuropathy has neuropathic pain (injury to the nerve system), but because they have had this neuropathic pain for so many years and it has already sensitized their pain system, they also have nociplastic pain.

Treating the neuropathic pain will be difficult when the whole pain system is sensitized, but eliminating the nociplastic pain can be quicker.

You will feel much more in control of your pain when you are able to remove the nociplastic element of your pain. Your quality of life will also improve because you will feel less anxious and fearful of the pain.

Many patients have told me that removing one component of their pain has made their lives much more manageable and predictable. They are able to reduce painkillers, start planning for their future and return to activities that they have not been able to do for many years. The residual pain is much easier to treat when the fog of nociplastic pain is lifted.

Acknowledging you have nociplastic pain

When a person doesn't recognize they have nociplastic pain, or they don't believe they can do anything about it or they are not ready to tackle it, that is a big obstacle.

If a patient with nociplastic pain refuses to accept the diagnosis, I find it very difficult to treat their other kinds of pains, nociceptive or neuropathic. Once a person acknowledges their nociplastic pain, and engages in brain retraining, it is much easier to treat nociceptive or neuropathic pain.

As we saw in the chapter *What Is Pain?* nociplastic pain, or sensitization, is like having a malfunctioning alarm in your home. Every time the alarm goes off, you call emergency services. The firefighters tell you over and over that there is no fire. But instead, every time the alarm goes off, you worry that there might be a real fire and you call emergency services again. Over and over. You need to believe it is a false alarm and understand that you should be calling the alarm company instead.

PRO TIP

If you do not acknowledge that you have a malfunction of your pain system, then you cannot retrain your pain system.

Our health system tends to medicalize problems, trying to find a body part that is broken and should be fixed. It neglects the obvious truth that the body is controlled by the mind, and that the mind is capable of creating bodily symptoms — and the mind can also remove bodily symptoms.

So, how do you know if you are ready to embark on retraining your brain? How do you know which stage you are at? There are a few questions that can help you find out.

Pain Stages of Change

PRECONTEMPLATION

↓

CONTEMPLATION

↓

ACTION

↓

MAINTENANCE

Prochaska and DiClemente published a seminal paper in 1983 about the four stages of change. They studied 872 subjects who changed their smoking habits on their own. They identified people in four different stages of readiness, which they called precontemplation, contemplation, action and maintenance.

PRECONTEMPLATION: The person is not even aware they have a problem.

CONTEMPLATION: The person recognizes they have a problem and they are aware of the need to be retrained.

ACTION: The person starts implementing the plan.

MAINTENANCE: The person maintains the changes and tries to prevent a relapse to the previous state.

Fast forward 40 years later and now we have more data to tell us what makes a person to move from one category to the next. It is education, information, data and testimonials.

The hardest and most difficult change is from precontemplation to contemplation. Once a person reaches the contemplation stage, they change their beliefs, actions and behaviors very quickly. But there is a big, tall, thick wall between precontemplation and contemplation.

What stage are you in?

In 1997, Kerns and colleagues (1997) published a questionnaire to apply to people with chronic pain. (Their model was adapted from smoking cessation to pain management.)

The full questionnaire has 30 statements, and I won't ask you to do them all. They range from "The best thing I can do is find a doctor who can figure out how to get rid of my pain once and for all" to "I am testing out some coping skills to manage my pain better."

PRADEEP IS STUCK IN THE PRECONTEMPLATION STAGE

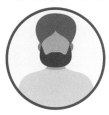 Pradeep was 45 years old when he had an injury at work. He required many months of physiotherapy, pain medications and counseling. He was referred to me two years later because his pain was not improving and he had not been able to return to work. His wife and their two kids had left him because he was angry, verbally abusive and had started drinking. His diet consisted of potato chips and soda, he had gained weight, was tired during the day and had insomnia at night.

His doctor prescribed opioids for pain, antidepressants for low mood, cannabis for insomnia, benzodiazepines for anxiety, muscle relaxants for tension and anti-inflammatories for his various joint pains.

I gave him the Pain Stages of Change Questionnaire. He was focused on finding a cure for his pain. He wanted me to order another MRI, in addition to the previous seven MRIs he had already done, plus many other diagnostic tests that were all inconclusive. He was precontemplating a change.

I examined him and told him that his body had healed perfectly, but now he had sensitization of the pain system. The alarm system of his body was hypervigilant, and he had developed fear of movement and fear of pain itself. He had nociplastic pain but he was not ready to accept it. It can be hard for many people in pain to be told that their pain is in part caused by fear.

Unfortunately, Pradeep did not accept my suggestions and he never came back to see me. If Pradeep had dealt with "the mountain" earlier, many of his problems would not have happened, and he would probably be in the maintenance stage now. Getting stuck in the first stage did not make Pradeep's mountain disappear. Instead, the mountain got bigger. Instead of just a mountain of pain, now his mountain had resentment, anger, broken relationships, loneliness, alcohol abuse, dependence on drugs and financial strains.

If you are interested, you can find a link to the full version in the *References and Resources* section at the end of this book. I would like you to read three statements in the last category, the category of people who are in the maintenance stage:

☑ "I have learned some good ways to keep my pain problem from interfering with my life."

☑ "When my pain flares up, I find myself automatically using coping strategies that have worked in the past."

☑ "I use what I have learned to help keep my pain under control." (Kerns et al., 1997)

My hope is that by the end of this book you will answer "yes" to all these statements. This, for me, is the perfect example of conquering your pain.

Moving from precontemplation to maintenance

It can take great courage to get beyond the precontemplation stage. But moving forward is key to making progress. I have found that the chances of treatment success are much smaller among patients who are in the precontemplation stage. We need to spend time moving them to the next stage, contemplation. Once they reach that stage, they progress quickly to the next stage, action, and then maintenance.

Once a person tastes the freedom that comes when they do not fear the pain anymore, they realize how much progress they can make. Many also have other challenges, such as anger and substance-use disorders, that keep their brain hostage to pain. (We talk more about these subjects in the next chapter.) Once people recognize that they can make a change, they usually regret all the moments they have lost in their lives by not participating in family celebrations, community gatherings, trips and parties.

If you are in the contemplation or action stages, keep reading this book! You will enjoy making progress, and then you will want to tell your story to other people who are in the precontemplation stage.

If you are in the maintenance stage, congratulations! You should tell your story to inspire others.

> I would love to hear which stage you are at.
> Tag me on social media using this hashtag:
> #ConquerPainWithDrFurlan

Rewiring Your Neuronal Pathways

Retraining the pain system involves wiring new neuronal pathways. That is how we learn new things.

When we are born, we don't know how to walk, talk, feed ourselves, read or do other complex tasks such as drive a car and talk at the same time. We learn by practicing. When neurons are activated, they fire an electrical impulse. When two neurons fire together, they wire together — this means they form a new synapse. A synapse is a connection between two neurons.

> Neurons that fire together wire together. You can rewire the connections in your pain system.

NEUROPLASTICITY

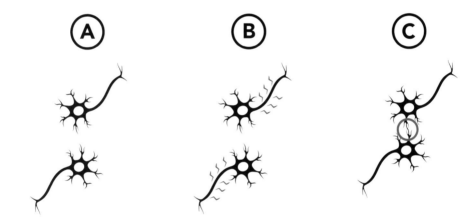

A Two neurons

B Two neurons firing together

C Two neurons wiring together. A synapse between two neurons is formed.

"Once a person tastes the freedom that comes when they do not fear the pain anymore, they realize how much progress they can make."

How chronic pain wires new synapses: three short stories

If you have chronic pain, then your brain has created many new synapses. The short case studies here provide a few examples.

KYLE AND THE CAR SEAT

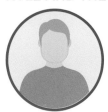

Kyle had low back pain. In the beginning, his pain was aggravated by sitting in the front seat of his car. His brain created a connection between that car seat and the pain. Now, even years after his low back pain has resolved, that synapse is still alive and well. Every time Kyle sits in the front seat of a car, his brain receives a pain signal. The pain is not coming from the lower back area. It is coming from the memory created by that synapse.

LISA AT HER SON'S HOUSE

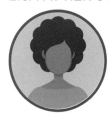

Lisa has hip arthritis. She lives in a two-storey house. The pain is worse when she goes up and down stairs. When she is at her son's house taking care of her grandchildren, she can go up and down without any pain. Her brain created a connection between her house's staircase and her pain. The pain is not coming from her hips; otherwise, she would feel pain at her son's house too.

PATRICIA AND THE PAVLOVIAN CONDITIONING REFLEX

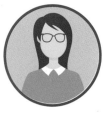

Patricia used opioids to treat her neck pain for more than 10 years. She felt 95 percent better immediately after putting the tablet in her mouth. This doesn't make sense, because the opioid pill needs to be swallowed, digested in the stomach and metabolized in the liver before it can activate the pain receptors in the brain. The fact that she felt much better just by putting the tablet in her mouth showed that her brain created a connection between the tablet in the mouth and pain relief. This is what we call a Pavlovian reflex, or classical conditioning. Ivan Pavlov demonstrated that dogs started salivating even before their food arrived because they were conditioned.

Ten Practices to Retrain Your Pain System

All of the connections your brain has created when you have chronic pain can be undone. We need to use brain exercises to disconnect these neurons. I call this physiotherapy for the brain.

Retraining your pain system is not complicated. The following suggestions will get you started.

The first three practices are key to opening your mind to the possibility that your pain is nociplastic and that it will get better with rewiring the connections in your pain system.

The next three practices direct you not to diagnose yourself and to get professional advice.

The last four practices are essential for you to follow to maintain the "rewiring" of your pain system. They will help to keep you motivated, especially when you experience a flare-up or another acute pain condition.

> Pain reprocessing is like physiotherapy for the brain.

1. *Make sure you understand what nociplastic pain is.* If you need to, reread the chapter *What Is Pain?*

2. *Watch my YouTube video* about central sensitization.

3. *Read books* about brain retraining, reprocessing neural networks, neuroplasticity, reprograming, unlearning pain memories and so on. Consult the list of suggested resources at the end of this book.

4. *Confirm with your doctor that you have nociplastic pain.* Don't try to self-diagnose. Ask if you have chronic pain in the sense that it is a malfunctioning of the pain system. But be mindful that there are many clinicians out there who have never heard of nociplastic pain, central sensitization or malfunctioning of the pain system. These are fairly recent concepts. If your doctor or therapist is one of these, tell them to read this book.

5. *Talk to your physiotherapist about fear of movement and fear of pain.* A physiotherapist will probably have longer appointments than doctors have, so you can have a longer discussion with them. Movement is one of the best therapies we know to retrain the brain. We will talk about that in *Step 7: Make Room in Your Toolbox.*

WATCH MY VIDEO ON CENTRAL SENSITIZATION

6 *Ask a psychologist or mental health counselor to help you* with emotional problems that could be predisposing your pain system to be sensitized. Start mind-body therapies as soon as possible. Some of them are free online or via apps for smartphones. We will talk about these in *Step 2: Control Your Emotions*.

7 *Join a peer group* of people with chronic pain who are in the maintenance stage. We will talk about this in *Step 5: Get Help from Others*. These can be online, social media or in-person groups. Don't join groups of people who are pre-contemplators. They are still looking for a quick fix and they don't have the answers you need.

8 *Practice some mind-body exercises* on your own. I will describe my favorites in this chapter.

9 *Seek out testimonials* from people who have overcome their chronic pain with brain retraining. Check the link, left, for my video with a successful patient.

10 *Keep reading this book with an open mind.* Remember that I am writing this book because I've seen people succeed at conquering chronic pain with brain retraining over and over. I know it is possible. I know you can do it. You must be very motivated, or else you would not have come so far in this book.

WATCH MY VIDEO INTERVIEW WITH A CHRONIC PAIN PATIENT

"I've seen people succeed at conquering chronic pain with brain retraining over and over. I know it is possible. I know you can do it."

Are you ready to sign this contract?

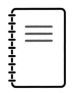

Let's do an exercise. If you have nociplastic pain, I want you to commit to retraining your pain system.

How do you start retraining your pain system? It is not magic or a secret therapy. It is quite simple. Anyone can do it, no matter what your educational background or socio-economic status.

All you need is to want it. That is why I'm asking you to write and sign this contract between you and yourself.

1 Get out your journal. Use the contract below as your model.

I _____ (your name) understand that my pain is a consequence of the alarm system of my body that is malfunctioning. That although I feel pain in my _____ (write the body part that hurts), the origin of my pain is not there, it is in the system that interprets the pain, and this system is located in my brain. I do not need any diagnostic image, or blood test to find out what the cause of my pain is. I commit to retraining my pain system to feel normal pain again and to eliminate my fear of pain.

_____ (your signature) _____ / _____ / _____ (today's date)

PS: This agreement is between you and yourself. Please do not send it to me or to your doctor.

Congratulations! You have just taken the most important step toward conquering your chronic pain.

This step is like placing your order to buy mountain climbing equipment. Once you press the payment button on your order, you have made the decision to climb the mountain. Now that you've paid, you must go. You don't want to waste your investment, and if you give up, you will get nothing in return.

Mind-Body Exercises to Retrain the Pain System

Below are examples of some of my favorite mind-body exercises that will help you to retrain your pain system. I recommend you seek professional help to identify which of these exercises are best suited for you. A variety of free resources available on the Internet offer these exercises. There are also many paid apps, books and groups that will guide you in doing these exercises.

Yoga

Yoga is a practice that focuses on the connections between mind and body. It uses posture, meditations and breathing exercises. Recent scientific studies have shown that practicing yoga has the opposite effect of pain on the brain. For example, the size of the insula (a part of the brain that is involved in pain tolerance) is increased as a result of regular yoga practice. It seems that yoga shifts the brain from a flight or fight response (sympathetic system) to a rest and heal state (parasympathetic system) (Villemeure, 2015).

Graded motor imagery

Graded motor imagery (GMI) includes three techniques: left/right discrimination training, explicit motor imagery and mirror therapy (Moseley, 2005). This approach has been demonstrated in various randomized controlled trials of patients with complex regional pain syndrome (CRPS) and phantom limb pain (pain from a limb that is no longer there).

PRO TIP

Professional athletes use explicit motor imagery as training for mastering their abilities. You can use it to retrain your brain by imagining movement without pain.

- An important part of retraining the brain involves a person's ability to identify left or right images of their painful body part(s). In *left/right discrimination training,* you are presented with a series of cards showing pictures of body parts and you have to identify if that picture represents a left or right body part.
- After that, you move on to *explicit motor imagery,* which includes thinking about moving without actually moving. The use of imagined movements can be painful. By imagining movements, you use the same areas of the brain as you would use if you were actually doing the movements. Professional athletes use this technique as training for mastering their abilities.

- Finally, in **mirror therapy,** you use a mirror to fool the brain. For example, you place your affected arm in front of your body, but your eyes are actually seeing a reflection of your other, healthy arm. When you exercise the affected side, your brain sees the good side moving. In that way, your brain is trained to accept that the affected side is not so bad.

Graded sensorimotor retraining

This new intervention is designed to demonstrate to the brain that moving the lower back area is not harmful, even though a person feels pain when they do these movements. Participants learn that the more they move, the more conditioned their bodies get, the stronger their muscles become, and they can actually perform many activities they weren't able to do before.

In a 2022 randomized trial of 276 people with chronic low back pain, a 12-week program of graded sensorimotor retraining significantly reduced pain intensity (Bagg et al., 2022). That treatment involved:

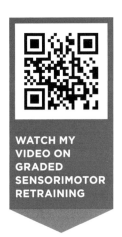

WATCH MY VIDEO ON GRADED SENSORIMOTOR RETRAINING

- Pain education about the neuroscience of pain
- Sensory retraining and imagining movements of the lower back area
- Experiencing movements of the lower back area and reframing them as non-dangerous movements

Somatic tracking

Somatic tracking has three components: mindfulness, safety reappraisal and positive affect induction. This approach has been proven effective in a randomized controlled trial for patients with chronic low back pain (Ashar, 2021).

1. **Mindfulness** is used to explore pain sensations with a sense of objective interest and curiosity. Being mindful means you notice the sensation just as a biological event, without having to change it, explain it or get rid of it.

2. **Safety reappraisal** takes the form of affirmations that these sensations are not harmful. You or your therapist can affirm that the sensation you feel are real but they are not a signal that there is anything broken or diseased. You keep repeating that you are "safe" and the body part that hurts is "safe" and is "perfectly healthy" — until you believe it. You teach your mind that your brain is simply

misinterpreting the signals coming from that body part as dangerous. You say "My spine is strong and healed. I can do anything I want. I don't have restrictions."

③ With **positive affect induction**, a therapist will use positive words and humor to lighten the mood and help you see the sensation as an observer would. Whatever happens to the sensation is acceptable. It can get worse or better. It doesn't matter because now you know it is safe and that there is nothing broken, which means that using that body part will not cause any harm.

Six Rs to unlearn pain

This program has been coined as a method to "unlearn pain" by Dr. Howard Schubiner (2010). The components of the program are the six Rs:

① **Reading** about mind-body syndrome

② **Repudiation** of the physical explanations for the symptoms

③ **Writing** exercises

④ **Reflecting** with meditative exercises

⑤ **Reprogramming** the mind

⑥ **Rebuilding** your life

The first step involves gaining knowledge about mind-body connections and convincing yourself that the only explanation for your pain is the mind-body connection and that you can be helped by this program. The second step is to reject any diagnoses for your symptoms that have been given by doctors who are unfamiliar with the mind-body syndrome. The remaining steps are designed to activate the conscious portions of your mind to help you to unlearn your pain. This process can be quick for some people, but for others, it may take several weeks to months.

Empowered relief

Empowered relief consists of a single-session, two-hour pain class that includes pain neuroscience education, mindfulness principles and cognitive behavioral therapy (CBT) skills to identify distressing thoughts and emotions, cognitive reframing, a relaxation response exercise and a self-soothing action plan.

Participants in this class receive a 20-minute relaxation audio file with binaural tones. Binaural tones, or beats, are created by two separate microphones to record the sounds, and these sounds are played separately to each ear. They activate the left and right brain hemisphere at different rhythms and pitches. They can strengthen brain waves and may have an influence on emotions and thoughts.

In a randomized trial published by Darnall and colleagues (2021), they showed that eight sessions of empowered relief with CBT helped people to reduce some unhelpful thoughts like catastrophization (imagining the worst), and also reduced the intensity of pain they were feeling. It also helped them to be more physically active and socially engaged.

Eye movement desensitization and reprocessing

Some people have nociplastic pain because of emotional trauma in their past, including various psychological stressors. We will talk more about these stressors in the next chapter.

Retraining the pain pathways also involves resolving those emotional traumas. **Eye movement desensitization and reprocessing** (EMDR) is a type of brain retraining that uses eye movements and memory of distressing events. This treatment was developed by Francine Shapiro in the 1980s. The person is asked to recall distressing experiences while moving their eyes side to side or tapping either side of their body.

EMDR is a way of reprocessing traumatic memories inside the memory networks of the brain, which contain related thoughts, images, emotions and sensations. When a distressing or traumatic memory is not properly processed, the distorted thoughts, images, emotions and perceptions are not stored adequately and the person experiences them as vivid and current events. The purpose of eye movements is to provide an external stimulus while the person is focusing on an internal distressing memory.

Next Steps

The exercises described above offer various approaches to retraining your pain system. Remember to ask your doctor or pain clinician what they recommend for you. We will look at some other options for mind-body exercises and therapies to help you with your emotions in the next chapter, *Step 2: Control Your Emotions.*

Are there any reasons why someone should not retrain their pain system?

There are no contraindications to retraining the pain system. At most, what can happen is that the person will regulate their emotions around the painful sensations, they will fear less when pain is present, they will request fewer painkillers, and there will be fewer unnecessary visits to doctors, hospitals, pain clinics, emergency departments and fewer diagnostic tests.

Retraining the pain system will reduce the sensitization and amplification of pain in the brain. As a result, it will help with sleep quality, concentration, mood and anxiety.

When someone has mixed types of pains, nociplastic pain is like a loud noise in the room that does not allow the people to have a normal conversation or to listen to music. It is very hard to diagnose and treat nociceptive or neuropathic pain when there is a large contribution from nociplastic pain.

How long will it take to retrain my brain?

This is will depend on many factors. In some people it will be fast, but for others, it may take years. It depends on how long the person has had chronic pain, the previous treatments and diagnoses the person received and the messages the person has heard from the other clinicians. It will depend on their emotional state and if they have another psychological or psychiatric condition that needs to be adequately addressed.

The important message is that if this doesn't work for you, it may be that this is not the right time for you. You may come back to this type of retraining the pain system later.

Do I need to stop all other treatments I am taking in order to start retraining my pain system?

No, you don't need to stop any treatment you are currently taking for chronic pain. You can add retraining of the pain system to any treatment regimen you are receiving.

CONCLUSION

In this chapter we looked at why and how we can retrain our pain system. It is crucial that you are willing to give your best to retrain your pain system, because nobody else can do this for you. I use a holistic approach to treat the person who has pain, not just the pain that the person has. You should do the same.

KEY POINTS TO REMEMBER

- Eliminating nociplastic pain can be quicker and easier than eliminating other kinds of pain.
- Eliminating or reducing nociplastic pain helps to lessen other kinds of pain.
- Getting a diagnosis and being ready to make a change in your life are important steps to success in conquering pain.
- Chronic pain changes your brain, and retraining your pain system means wiring new neuronal pathways in your brain.
- There are steps you can take to retrain your pain system, including doing your research, consulting with others and making a contract with yourself.
- Consider the various mind-body exercises and approaches to brain retraining that are available. Many of them have been proven effective in reducing nociplastic pain.

LOOKING AHEAD

The pain system is not just the brain. It includes another very important system in our body: our emotional system, or the psychological state of our mind. In the next chapter, we will consider our emotions, and how they shape the way we feel and how we express pain.

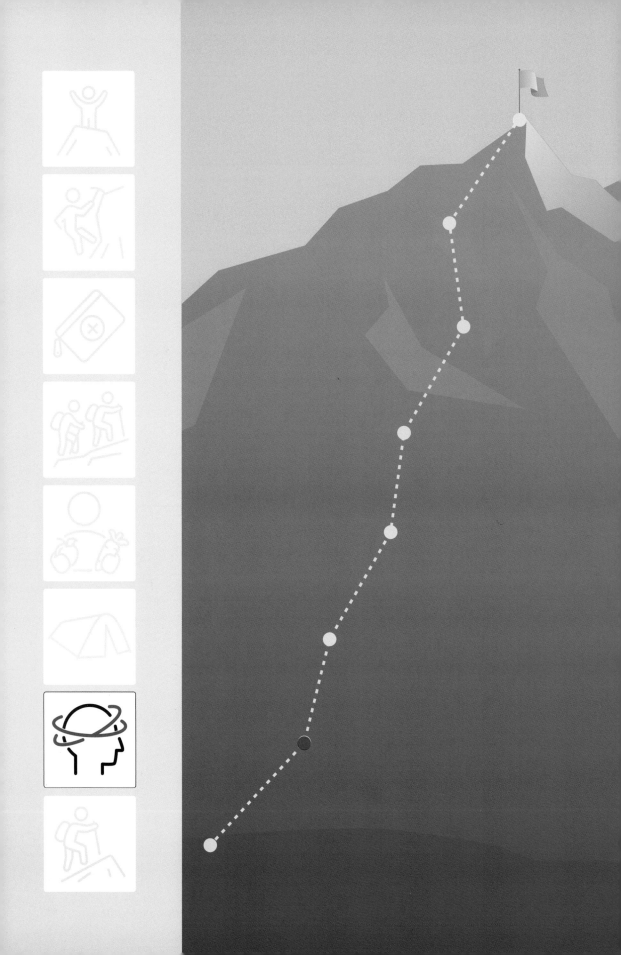

Control Your Emotions

The mountaineer will need to spend equal amounts of time preparing emotionally and physically, starting many months before their journey. They may even need to take a climbing course and provide evidence of their training and readiness to prove that they are prepared.

> **THE CLIMBING CODE**
> "Climb if you will, but remember that courage and strength are naught without prudence, and that a momentary negligence may destroy the happiness of a lifetime. Do nothing in haste; look well to each step, and from the beginning think what may be the end."
>
> — Edward Whymper (1871)

Have you ever noticed that some emotions are not helpful? Healthy people sometimes feel sad or frustrated, but people with chronic pain seem to be sad, frustrated, pessimistic, and/or angry more often than not.

"You need emotional control to conquer any challenge. There is no big or small mountain. Every mountain is a mountain."

In this chapter, I will help you to identify some emotions that are unhealthy and interfere with your journey to conquer chronic pain. Together we will explore some of these emotions and what to do about them.

You will learn why people with chronic pain have higher rates of unhealthy emotions. We will look at the most common types of emotional problems that affect people with chronic pain: anger, fear, depression and substance use. And we will discuss what you can do to prevent and to manage these emotional problems.

Learning about Emotions Is Essential to Conquering Pain

Don't skip this chapter. You are probably thinking "My pain is not psychological, so this does not apply to me." How can I convince you to read this full chapter? Let me try.

There is a reason why I placed this topic near the base of the mountain. I am not a literal mountain climber. But I have climbed many other mountains in my life, and I can assure you that the most important factor in succeeding at a challenge is your mindset. If you don't put your energy into that challenge, you will not be able to overcome it. You will give up early.

You need emotional control to conquer any challenge. There is no big or small mountain. Every mountain is a mountain.

Don't stop here! You are just starting to prepare mentally for climbing the chronic pain mountain.

By saying you need to prepare mentally, I am not saying that you are imagining your pain, faking it or that you don't have a physical problem. Everyone needs to learn emotional control. If you let your emotions control you, you will not be able to do what I will ask you to do in the next chapters.

So keep reading.

Your mind is your most potent weapon against chronic pain. Still, many people neglect it, including some of my colleague physicians. There is a tendency to look for and find a biological cause for all pains, and fix them with drugs, injections and surgeries.

On the other hand, there are a lot of scams and fake theories about the power of the mind. We must be wary of the multitude of useless ideas and products that are promoted and sold offering a quick fix to the mind problem.

There is also a lot of research incentive to conduct trials of drugs, injections and surgeries, but very little on mind-body therapies or self-management strategies.

The research-proven evidence to back up mind-body therapies for chronic pain is much stronger and more convincing than the evidence for any drug, injection or surgery. Still, that knowledge is not taught in medical schools, and many patients are cheated by a healthcare system that provides drugs and interventions and not mind-body therapies, which can be much less expensive and do not require sophisticated equipment.

> **Our mind tells us what we feel, what we think, what we remember and what we want**

The mind is where our feelings, thoughts, memories and desires are processed. Our mind tells us what we feel, what we think, what we remember and what we want.

MIND

Perceptions and feelings	"I feel"
Thoughts	"I think"
Memories	"I remember"
Desires	"I want"

We feel pain, we think about pain, we remember pain and we want pain to go away. Unfortunately, the more we think about pain, the more memory we create in our mind, and the harder it is to get rid of those memories. We need to learn how not to think about pain and how to distract our minds with other, more interesting things.

There is research showing that our emotions determine how much pain we feel. This means that the same painful stimulus or injury will seem worse, or more intense, when we are sad, and it will seem less intense when we are happy. If our brain is distracted with other tasks, we may be less aware of our pain than if our attention is focused on it, especially if we are frightened or angry about the pain.

Our brain may also get overwhelmed with feeling pain all the time and stay in a constant state of hypervigilance, always on the alert for even the tiniest sign of pain. This is very common with some chronic pain syndromes such as complex regional pain syndrome (CRPS), fibromyalgia and migraine.

There are aspects of our personalities, the way we were raised as a child and previous experiences in our lives, that make us all different. These differences also affect how we perceive, how we communicate and how we cope with pain.

Optimists tend to recover better from acute pain. They are also less likely to develop chronic pain, and if they do, it is not so debilitating. Catastrophizers are more likely to develop chronic pain and to suffer more from their pain.

For example, some people are more optimistic in general; they are the kind of people who are able to always see the bright side of things in life. They always imagine the best possible scenario of an action or an event. We know that people who have this kind of personality tend to recover better from acute pain. They are also less likely to develop chronic pain, and if they do, it is not so debilitating.

On the other hand, people who imagine the worst possible scenario of an action or an event and always worry that a catastrophe is going to happen are more likely to develop chronic pain and to suffer more from their pain.

"The more we think about pain, the more memory we create in our mind, and the harder it is to get rid of those memories."

The Conscious and Unconscious Mind

In simple terms, our mind has two levels: the conscious and the unconscious. The conscious mind contains the feelings, thoughts, memories and desires that we are aware of. It is our rational thinking, and we are able to talk about it, explain it and defend it. It is usually socially acceptable.

The unconscious mind contains the feelings, thoughts, memories and desires that we are not aware of. Much of this content is unacceptable or unpleasant, and it contrasts with and contradicts what our conscious mind would agree on and approve.

In his seminal book *The Mindbody Prescription* (1999), Dr. John Sarno explains that physical pain is a manifestation of an unconscious symptom that the conscious mind is trying to suppress or avoid. Therefore, pain becomes a distraction to suppress the rage of the unconscious mind.

HOW THE CONSCIOUS AND UNCONSCIOUS MINDS WORK

YOUR CONSCIOUS MIND ...	YOUR UNCONSCIOUS MIND ...
tells you that you are a good person	tells you that you are worthless and useless
tells you that you need to exercise and eat healthier	sabotages all your intentions to exercise and tempts you with junk food
tells you that you are lucky to get this job, while so many people are unemployed	tells you that you hate this job, you hate your boss and you don't want to work there anymore
tells you that your surgery went well, the surgeons did everything they could do to help you after your accident and you are happy they saved your life	tells you that the doctors were incompetent and they didn't care if you would end up with this chronic pain
tells you that you have already had enough lab tests, imaging studies, injections and surgeries for this chronic pain	keeps telling you that you still haven't found the right doctor, the one who will find something that is broken in your body and magically fix it

Your Mind Interprets Your Pain

> The mind is both capable of creating symptoms and capable of erasing symptoms.

Why are these two levels of our mind, conscious and unconscious, important to pain? Because our mind is where pain is interpreted and given meaning. Therefore, whatever is in the conscious or unconscious mind will interfere, very profoundly, with pain. Our mind can affect the intensity and quality of our pain, the suffering we feel because of that pain and our memories and feelings about our pain.

You don't need to spend time and money in years of psychotherapy to acknowledge that the mind is very powerful and has an influence on us. The mind is both capable of creating symptoms and capable of erasing symptoms.

> **You cannot block or separate the sensations you feel from your mind**

There is no way to separate the mind from pain. All sensations that we feel from any part of our body are carried to the brain, and the brain gives the final verdict on how it will react.

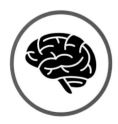

The brain will connect the dots ·········⟩ INCOMING SENSATION + EMOTIONS + MEMORY + ENVIRONMENT + WHO IS AROUND + FUTURE PREDICTIONS

If the mind decides that the sensation is not relevant and should be ignored, then the person will not interpret that sensation as pain. On the other hand, if the mind decides that the sensation is dangerous, it will interpret it as pain. The alarm goes off and makes a lot of noise.

How emotions create painful symptoms

The following two case studies show how fear, activated in the amygdala, causes "danger alerts," which in turn result in pain.

SARA AND HER STAGE FRIGHT

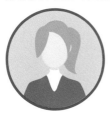

Sara had a fear of speaking in public. Stage fright is a common type of anxiety. The origin of the problem is fear. When she faced a situation in which she needed to go on a stage and speak, she had nausea, vomiting, abdominal pain, diarrhea, headache, shortness of breath and palpitations.

Sara didn't have a stomach infection, a lung problem or heart disease. She was having symptoms in her body, but they were created in her mind for a single purpose. The amygdala detected danger and it was trying to stop her from going on the stage, a situation identified as dangerous.

Once Sara recognized the source of her symptoms was her anxiety, she was able to reduce her fear and speak in public.

CARLOS AND HIS MORNING MEETINGS

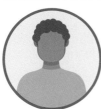

Carlos is a perfectionist. He grew up earning straight As, and he has won many medals and awards. He works at a financial company where his job is very demanding and stressful. Every morning he has a business meeting where he is questioned, and he believes he must have answers for everything. He dreaded these meetings. Some of the participants were very disrespectful and demeaning.

Carlos had headaches every morning. By noon they were better, but he was constantly fatigued and had difficulty concentrating. His amygdala had detected that the morning meetings were dangerous and was trying to keep Carlos from attending them. In case you are wondering, Carlos didn't have those headaches on weekends.

After Carlos realized that his headaches were stress-related, he learned relaxation and breathing techniques that included visualizations, parasympathetic activation and self-hypnosis. Now his headaches are gone.

> *Pain is in the brain. It is a construct of the mind.*
>
> Pain is an opinion about what is happening in the body. It is an interpretation of various sensations.
>
> The problem is, when we try to teach this to our patients, they think we are saying that their pain is not real, that they are faking it. Then they resist the idea and stop any attempt to learn these concepts.

There is no way to separate the mind from pain.

The main function of the pain system is to detect danger. The pain system is the alarm system of the body. But it can malfunction and it can be deceiving.

I'd like to return to my comparison of your pain system and a home alarm system.

THE SMOKE DETECTOR OF A HOUSE CAN BE TRIGGERED BY:

A dangerous fire in the house ⟶ a very good reason to call emergency services ✓

Someone preparing dinner and generating smoke ⟶ not a good reason to call emergency services ✗

A match or candle that is lighted very close to the sensor ⟶ a very bad reason to call emergency services ✗

If the mind, conscious or unconscious, does not feel safe, then a harmless sensation may be interpreted as pain.

So, what is the solution? There is no pill, manual therapy, physical exercise, surgery, injection or nerve block that will alleviate emotional pain. The only way to make the emotional pain go away is to go to the root cause of the problem, which could be related to your feelings, thoughts, memories or desires.

A mental health therapist specializing in mind-body therapies can help you to identify these abnormalities and how to eliminate or manage them. (Some examples of these therapies are included later in this chapter.)

What are you feeling?

Let's do an exercise. If you are a person with chronic pain, you may be having sensations of pain in various parts of your body.

1 Think about what you are feeling right now. Get your journal and record the emotions that you have related to your pain.

2 If you don't have pain right now, can you remember the last time that you had pain? For example, if you burned a finger on the stove, did you get angry because you forgot to put on the oven mitts? Write down your feelings and emotions related to that pain.

Here are some examples of unhealthy feelings or emotions

- Afraid
- Angry
- Devalued
- Forgotten
- Guilty
- Helpless
- Hopeless
- Lonely
- Lost
- Rejected
- Sad
- Stressed
- Tired
- Unsafe
- Weak
- Worried
- Worthless

Remember, you can only name these emotions if you are aware of them. But there might be feelings that are buried in your unconscious, which your mind is suppressing or repressing because they may not be acceptable to you or to the society where you live. These unconscious feelings also affect your health.

Some people may need to see a psychotherapist to get help with these feelings and emotions. They may be unable to get help by themselves. If this is your case, please get professional help now. Talk to your doctor and ask for a referral to a psychiatrist, a psychologist or a mental health counselor.

WHAT ARE YOU FEELING?

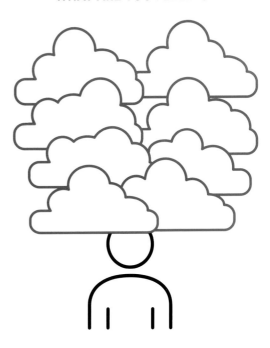

The Links between Sensations, Pain and Emotions

Unhealthy emotions may not be a direct consequence of being in constant pain. They may be what is perpetuating the pain itself.

People with chronic pain have a much higher rate of unhealthy emotions. They tend to feel mistreated, ignored, indifferent, undervalued, isolated, misinterpreted and fatigued.

How can someone feel happy and enjoy life if they have pain all the time?

You may believe your unhealthy emotions are the natural consequences of having constant, ongoing pain. In fact, these emotions might be what is perpetuating the pain in your pain system. Yes, it may sound contradictory, but unhealthy emotions may not be a direct consequence of being in constant pain.

To understand this, you need to know how our sensory system works, that our body contains many different types of sensations and that these sensations are linked to emotions.

The sensory system

The sensory system is responsible for our interactions with the exterior environment: vision, hearing, taste, smell, balance, touch, heat and cold, and nociception. (We learned about nociception, which occurs when pain receptors called nociceptors are activated, in *What Is Pain?* on page 22.) Nociception is a type of sensation, but our body has many other sensations. All these sensations are interpreted in the brain.

Sensations are connected to the emotion centers of the brain (the limbic system) to give meaning to them. A sensation in itself is not good or bad, but the brain assigns meaning to it. Is a sensation harmful or helpful? Should I be worried or calm? The brain will decide.

Consider, for example, hearing. There are some types of music that make us happy and others that make us sad.

Olfactory sensations can also affect our emotions: some smells can make us feel happy, for example, a nice perfume, while spoiled food may make us feel disgusted.

Most of the time the sensation of pain will be interpreted as a hostile emotion. There is rarely a situation in which pain is linked to a happy emotion. A person feeling pain most likely will want the pain to go away, to put an end to an unfriendly feeling. Pain is designed to be nasty and relentless because its function is to alert us that something is broken or faulty.

If it was pleasant, we would not know that we should seek medical attention to fix an injury or damage to our body.

Feelings and emotions are tightly linked to pain in the brain. They share similar circuits and neurotransmitters.

In people with chronic primary pain, there may be no nociception activity, yet functional imaging of the brain shows that the pain centers in the brain are being activated and there is pain. (Look at the figure on page 32 to remind yourself how this works.)

We learned in a previous chapter that because of central sensitization, chronic pain may become a false alarm that still makes noise even when the injury has already been healed. The electrical impulses generated by central sensitization will arrive at the brain and the brain will activate emotions in the same way as if there was nociception. The brain doesn't know that the electrical impulse is being originated by an injury in the foot (for example) or a centrally sensitized synapse in the spinal cord. It reacts the same way: "Danger, danger, danger!"

In chronic pain, the brain interprets the feelings and emotions as if there is an ongoing acute injury or insult to the body. With nociplastic pain (see pages 28–38), the circuits in the brain do not know that the injury has already healed, and they continue activating the emotional system that regulates our feelings.

Not all chronic pain is a malfunctioning of the pain system, however. In some cases, the emotional reaction to chronic pain will be at a level that is expected for that type of injury. For example, a person with chronic neuropathic pain secondary to nerve damage will feel sad and discouraged. They may find psychological support with cognitive behavioral therapy very very helpful in coping with that pain the rest of their life.

If you understand these concepts, your journey to conquering pain will be much easier.

False alarm! Even when an injury is already healed, the circuits in the brain may continue activating the emotional system that regulates our feelings.

"With nociplastic pain, the circuits in the brain do not know that the injury has already healed, and they continue activating the emotional system that regulates our feelings."

This model, which shows that an **injury** leads to **pain,** and **pain** leads to an **emotion,** is not correct. For example:

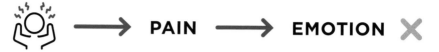

- The **injury** can be a fall, a car accident, a surgery or disk herniation in the spine.
- The **pain** can be a headache, a sore back, a tingling in the hand or a sciatica in the leg.
- The **emotion** could be anger, depression or anxiety.

The better explanation is that an **injury** leads to a **sensation,** which is the stimulation of sensory nerves that carry electrical impulses to the brain and tell the brain that something is wrong. (The technical name of the sensation is **nociception.** We introduced nociception on page 22 of *What Is Pain?*) And at the same time as the pain sensors (nociceptors) are activated, the emotional centers of the brain are activated.

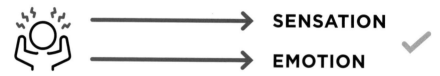

Now, we have multiple areas of the brain activated. The combination of the nociception sensations with emotions is what we call pain.

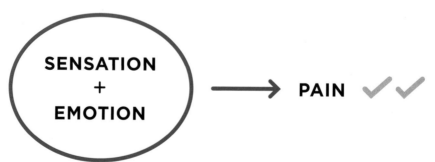

Both of these models are correct. Injuries or diseases lead to sensations and emotions. When we combine a sensation (like nociception) with an unpleasant emotion, we interpret it as pain. I'm not suggesting that you need to be happy when you feel pain. That would be masochism and that is an aberration.

Identifying Your Emotions

Earlier in this chapter, I asked you to name your emotions related to pain. Some common feelings among people with chronic pain are anger, fear, anxiety, depression, hopelessness, tiredness, loneliness and helplessness. They are valid and justified emotions. We will discuss some of these emotions in more detail. It is important to identify them as soon as they start.

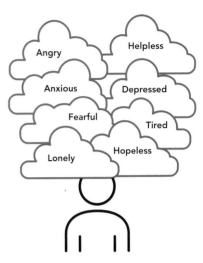

Once we identify them, it is even more important to eliminate any unhelpful emotions and thoughts before they affect other aspects of your health.

Memory of pain is a real condition and is the major driver of chronic primary pain, or nociplastic pain. Once the brain feels pain for a long time, it creates a memory. Even if the injury is healed, the pain is still felt by the brain.

GETTING PROFESSIONAL HELP

This chapter can assist you in identifying your emotions and considering if they are "as expected" for a person with chronic pain or if they are "out of proportion."

It is expected that a person living with constant pain may have abnormal emotions compared to a person who does not have ongoing daily pain. The problem is when these emotions are so out of proportion that they start interfering with the person's quality of life, controlling what they do or stop doing, blocking them from achieving their life's goals and dreams. This is the point where the emotion must be treated and the person may need professional help.

If this is your situation, you may need to see a psychologist, a counselor or a psychiatrist. There are many professionals who are trained in mental health disorders. They will help you to identify disturbed feelings or thoughts and will guide you in replacing them with helpful and constructive emotions and ideas. The sooner you get mental health support, the better. The longer you wait, the harder you and the therapist will have to work to treat your harmful feelings and thoughts and undo their consequences.

The field of psychology has made tremendous advances in the past decades and a great number of high-quality scientific studies have shown that it is possible to obtain good results for mental health conditions among people with chronic pain.

Our thoughts and emotions affect our behaviors, and our behaviors affect our thoughts and emotions. Our mind is where our thoughts, feelings, memories and desires are processed.

CASE STUDY

PATRICK FORGIVES AND FORGETS

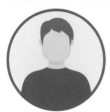 Patrick was 46 years old when he started coming to our clinic. When he was 35, he was involved in a car accident. His car was stopped at a traffic light, and another car hit him from behind. He sustained a whiplash injury (a neck problem caused by a rapid back-and-forth movement like the cracking of a whip). After that, he developed chronic neck pain, migraines and temporomandibular joint (TMJ) dysfunction.

The person who hit his car did not suffer any injury and lives a normal, happy life. Patrick was very angry at the other driver and felt a sense of injustice toward him. He also developed insomnia, high blood pressure, depression and anxiety in addition to the chronic neck pain and headaches.

Our team helped him to recognize that his anger was not helpful and that all that energy was harmful to his health. It would be better if he forgave and forgot the other driver and moved on with his life.

Initially Patrick did not accept our suggestion, but as time passed, his pain was not getting better and he started seeing a counselor for anger management. When he returned to see me, he was no longer angry at the other driver. He told us that he was able to manage his neck pain with stretches and mind-body relaxation techniques. He did not have any more headaches and was sleeping much better.

Anger

Anger is a strong feeling of displeasure or annoyance and often of active opposition to an insult, injury or injustice.

In clinical practice, we use a questionnaire called the Injustice Experience Questionnaire (IEQ-SF) (Sullivan et al., 2008). It has 12 statements, each one scored from 0, for never, to 4, all the time. The following three statements are examples from the IEQ-SF:

- "It all seems so unfair."
- "Nothing will ever make up for all that I have gone through."
- "I am troubled by fears that I may never achieve my dreams." (Sullivan et al., 2008)

Patrick, the patient I described above, had the highest score that I have ever seen in my clinic: 48 points.

Many trained mental healthcare professionals deliver anger management therapy, including psychologists, social workers and psychiatrists. Anger management therapy can be delivered individually or in a group. Options include acceptance and commitment therapy (ACT), cognitive behavioral therapy (CBT), mindfulness training and stress-reduction training.

What should I expect from anger management therapy?

Usually, the therapist will help you to identify unhelpful or negative thoughts or emotions. These thoughts generally follow certain patterns. They may ask you to imagine an incident that would provoke intense anger, and then you come up with strategies to identify that emotion and practice healthier coping mechanisms. The therapist will also help you to understand how anger has affected your relationships with other people around you, and how to restore those relationships.

We do not prescribe medication to manage anger issues if that is the only problem a person has. In some cases, anger is associated with other emotional disorders, for example, post-traumatic stress disorder (PTSD) or depression.

Fear is an unpleasant emotion or thought that you have when you are frightened or worried by something dangerous, painful or harmful that is happening or that might happen.

At the beginning of this chapter, I shared how Sara was affected by her fear of speaking in public and how Carlos suffered because he dreaded his morning meetings.

I see many patients who have chronic pain due to osteoarthritis, a degenerative disease of the cartilage of major joints that slowly causes deformities, pain and creaky joints. Below is a story about one such patient and her fears.

Fear is a natural reaction of our body. Fear protects us from threats by warning us to get ready to deal with a dangerous situation. I have already mentioned the amygdala. We are each born with this organ inside of our brain responsible for fear. Anxiety disorders are associated with hyperactivity of the amygdala. Examples of these disorders include generalized anxiety disorder (GAD), post-traumatic stress disorder (PTSD), obsessive-compulsive disorder (OCD), panic disorder, phobias and social anxiety disorder.

CASE STUDY

LUCY AND THE JOINT LUBRICANT

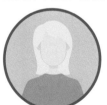 Lucy is an 80-year-old woman with osteoarthritis in almost every joint of her body. She was terrified of moving because her joints make a lot of noises when she moves, and she was afraid movement was aggravating her arthritis.

She came to me asking for "strong painkillers." I explained that the best painkiller for osteoarthritis is motion. Movement makes the joints produce more lubricant.

She enrolled in aqua fitness classes twice a week, then increased to three times a week, and she enjoyed it so much that she was doing five days a week. Her joints were still making noise, but she got stronger muscles, more range of motion, better balance and less pain.

Lucy never asked me for pain pills again. And she doesn't pay attention to the cracking sounds of her joints anymore.

Remember, pain is a sensation coupled with an emotion, and therefore the person with chronic pain may consequently develop fear associated with pain. These feelings are paralyzing, as they create a vicious cycle of fear, avoidance and additional pain due to deconditioning, weakness and lack of movement. The problem is that the person will avoid healthy activities if they are afraid that these activities will be painful. This avoidance coping strategy is harmful to the healing process, as the person will avoid moving, and movement is the best strategy for healing from acute injuries and preventing chronic pain.

DON'T FEED THE CYCLE OF FEAR-AVOIDANCE-PAIN

Two people may experience the same injury and have completely difference consequences. See the diagram below.

If you have no fear of movement, you will confront the problem and heal faster.

If you are afraid of movement and have negative thoughts and emotions, you will develop a fear of pain and pain anxiety. You will avoid activities that could potentially cause more pain but then, as a consequence, become more isolated, weak and depressed, and suffer from low self-esteem. Those emotions will accentuate the perception of pain, and that will feed the cycle of pain $\longrightarrow$ fear $\longrightarrow$ disuse $\longrightarrow$ more pain.

THE FEAR-AVOIDANCE-PAIN CYCLE

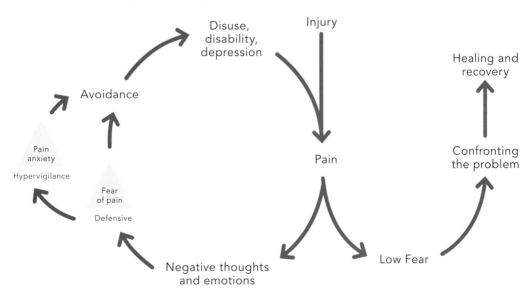

FEAR-AVOIDANCE BEHAVIORS

The sooner we identify fear-avoidance behaviors, the better.

When I suspect that my patient is having high fear-avoidance behaviors, I use a validated test called a Fear-Avoidance Beliefs Questionnaire created by Gordon Waddell and colleagues (1993).

This questionnaire was developed for low back pain patients. The authors of this questionnaire found that people with higher scores need to be supervised more than those with lower scores to prevent them from developing chronic low back pain.

There are two subset of questions, one that assesses fear related to physical activity, and the other about work-related activities. Each question is scored from 0, for completely disagree, to 6, for completely agree.

These are some examples of the questionnaire statements related to physical activity and to work:

- "Physical activity makes my pain worse."
- "I cannot do physical activities which (might) make my pain worse."
- "My work aggravated my pain."
- "I cannot do my normal work until my pain is treated." (Waddell et al., 1993)

PRO TIP

Check what high-performance athletes do. They don't fear pain; they confront pain with movement. As a consequence, they heal a lot faster. If a person gets stuck in fear and avoids movement, they will delay the recovery process and probably end up more disabled and depressed.

I spend a lot of time explaining to my patients that fear is unhelpful and paralyzing. It is an inadequate response and it will not protect them. You need to trust and believe that if you move, that will expedite your progress toward recovery.

The main barrier we face is that movement may initially aggravate pain. You need to feel worse before you feel better. But you will feel better if you move. When you feel pain after exercise, it can be because one of two possibilities:

- Muscle soreness: the pain we feel when we exercise a muscle that has not been used for a long time
- A malfunctioning pain system

The first does not require any special treatment; just wait 48 to 72 hours and the pain will go away. The second requires some modification in the exercise routine: instead of doing sporadic vigorous and fatiguing exercises, you need to do regular, daily, low-intensity and short-duration exercises, and increase the duration and intensity very gradually. (We discuss this more in *Step 7* on page 225.)

Anxiety is an uncomfortable feeling of nervousness or worry about something that is happening or might happen in the future.

While fear is related to something that is happening now, anxiety is an anticipation of something bad. It is future-oriented. Anxiety is a normal reaction of our mind and it stimulates us to take action or protect ourselves. If a student does not get anxious about an exam, she will not study for it.

STRESS AND RESILIENCE

Fear and anxiety are linked to the sympathetic nerve system (SNS), the part of your autonomic nerve system that is activated in the fight or flight response. The SNS will release adrenaline, noradrenaline and cortisol, which are the neurotransmitters and hormones of stress reactions.

Stress is any external force that causes a change in a substance. For example, if we apply too much pressure on a piece of metal, it will deform. Each material has a different resilience, depending on their composition. A material with a lot of resilience, like foam, will be able to return to its original form after being exposed to a lot of pressure, or stress. A metal plate will not return to its original form after being exposed to stress because it has low resilience.

The same concept applies to our mental state. A person with high levels of resilience is able to endure high-pressure, stressful situations and return to their previous mental state without much change. Another person with low levels of resilience will be changed by each stressful situation that life throws at them, and they will not be able to return to their original pre-stress state.

HOW DO WE DEVELOP RESILIENCE?

Resilience is not sold in a pill that you can swallow. And you will not become resilient by reading a book. Resilience is more than just a state of mind. It is a personality trait that is built over many years, starting from when we were inside our mother's womb. A pregnant woman who is having high levels of stress, fear and anxiety will pass that to the fetus.

PRO TIP

An athlete who is not anxious about competition will not give his best in training and at practices. The problem is when anxiety is out of proportion for a given circumstance.

ANTHONY, A TRUCK DRIVER WITH NECK PAIN

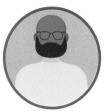

Anthony is a 31-year-old truck driver with neck pain. He came to my clinic because he had tried more than 10 different physiotherapists and chiropractors and nothing helped. He didn't want to take any painkillers as he was concerned that it would keep him from operating the 12-wheeler heavy cargo truck he drives for work.

His pain was constant, annoying and made him very impatient. He said his mood depended on how his neck was feeling, and that he didn't want to be rude to people, but sometimes he would explode in anger for no reason, just because he couldn't take the pain anymore.

We did some questionnaires and interviews and found that his pain was worse when he was worried about his marriage, his children and finances.

He did a few months of psychotherapy and he learned to identify the connection between his emotions and neck pain. He was able to soothe his pain by doing regular relaxation, body scans, meditations and mindfulness.

During the early years, mainly from birth to age six, the brain is still under development, and stressful situations such as neglect, abuse, parental separation, death of a parent, living with an adult who uses drugs or has psychiatric disease, all can affect the brain development and the centers of fear, emotions and resilience. (See adverse childhood experiences on pages 51–53.)

"We cannot avoid stressful situations in life, but we can control how they affect us."

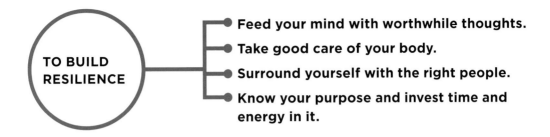

TO BUILD RESILIENCE
- Feed your mind with worthwhile thoughts.
- Take good care of your body.
- Surround yourself with the right people.
- Know your purpose and invest time and energy in it.

To build resilience, start from inside, with your thoughts, and move to the outside.

1. *Your thoughts:* Do you feed your mind with what is truly worthwhile, what is right, pure and proper? Don't feed your thoughts with junk. Did you accept the changes and challenges that were put in front of you during your life? Do you embrace rational or irrational thinking? If you are religious, read your sacred book a few times. Invest time in reading healthy literature and watching motivating speakers and videos.

2. *Your body:* Take good care of your body, including nutrition, sleep, exercise, relaxation and following medical advice.

3. *The people you surround yourself with:* Keep a small circle of about five people who are very close to you, who are understanding and empathetic. These are people who you can say anything to at any time. Keep a larger group of about 12 to 20 friends that you can see regularly and exchange ideas and have fun. There are also benefits to having a much larger social network of acquaintances, even if you know little about them other than their names (and they know very little about you). Invest time and energy in nurturing your small circle, but don't forget your friends too. The rest of the world? Don't worry about what they think or say about you.

4. *Your purpose:* Spend time doing some soul searching. Life is too short to spend without a purpose. Once you discover your purpose, invest time and energy writing your life goals, how you will help others and make this world a better place.

If you have pain, then feeling anxious about your future is an expected reaction. There is nothing wrong with that. The problem is how you respond to pain, which is a stressful situation. When pain comes back, you have a flare-up or the disease that caused your pain is getting worse, then it is time to practice, demonstrate and grow your resilience. Be sure to appreciate your strength, to celebrate your successes, and to love and care for yourself.

THERAPIES FOR RELAXATION AND ANXIETY

The therapist may use one of many kinds of therapy to help the person with anxiety disorders, including acceptance and commitment therapy (ACT), cognitive behavioral therapy (CBT), mindfulness-based stress reduction or breathing relaxation techniques.

HOW DO WE KNOW IF YOUR ANXIETY IS NORMAL OR EXCESSIVE?

There are many ways to measure if a person is too anxious. In the pain clinic, I use a questionnaire called Generalized Anxiety Disorder – 7 (GAD-7), created by R. Spitzer and colleagues (2006). It contains seven questions with possible answers from 0, for not at all, to 3, for nearly every day. The person is instructed to answer how often they have been bothered by the following over the past two weeks:

- "Feeling nervous, anxious or on the edge"

- "Not being able to stop or control worrying"

- "Worrying too much about different things"

- "Trouble relaxing"

- "Being so restless that it's hard to sit still"

- "Becoming easily annoyed or irritable"

- "Feeling afraid as if something awful might happen" (Spitzer et al., 2006)

Higher scores suggest a clinically significant anxiety disorder, such as generalized anxiety disorder, panic disorder, social phobia or PTSD. Then, the person needs a proper diagnosis, so we refer them to a psychiatrist, which is a physician specialist in mental health disorders. The psychiatrist may recommend mind-body therapies, medication or both.

Activation of the parasympathetic nervous system

The parasympathetic nervous system (PNS) is one of the two parts of the autonomic nervous system. It is the opposite of the sympathetic nervous system, which responds to stress by preparing the body for danger.

The PNS, which is responsible for the "rest and digest" functions, slows down your body's responses and helps to bring calm. When it is active, it constricts the pupils of your eyes, stimulates the production of saliva, and activates the vagus nerve, a long cranial nerve that contains motor and sensory fibers.

We have two vagus nerves, the right and the left. Each one exits the brain and controls the heart, the lungs, the esophagus, the stomach, the liver, pancreas, spleen, kidneys, adrenals, and intestines.

You can deliberately activate your parasympathetic nervous system. There are a number of ways to do this:

- Reduce the amount of stress you put on yourself. Reduce the news and social media you consume.
- Spend more time in mindful moments, like mindful eating, mindful walking, meditation, praying, gratitude, breathing, and contact with nature.
- Take time to do physical and mental exercises. Those are mind-body connections.
- Do vagus nerve exercises.
- Spend time laughing and socializing with friends.
- Sing or chant.
- Get a massage.
- Take a cold shower.

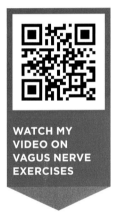

WATCH MY VIDEO ON VAGUS NERVE EXERCISES

FAQ

When do we use medications to treat anxiety disorders?

We prescribe medications to reduce anxiety symptoms mainly when they are affecting the patient's sleep or ability to carry out daily activities such as grooming, shopping, cooking, cleaning, bathing, working and socialization. Your doctor may prescribe one or more of certain antidepressants or gabapentinoids to treat anxiety. See *Step 6: Check Your Medicine Cabinet* for more about these medications.

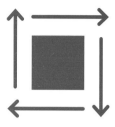

Square breathing relaxation exercise

I teach a breathing technique that can be done anywhere anytime. It is called square breathing. This technique activates the parasympathetic nervous system to relax the muscles and calm anxiety.

Use this breathing technique to help relieve anxiety.

1 Breathe in for 4 seconds.

2 Hold your breath for 4 seconds.

3 Breathe out for 4 seconds.

4 Hold for 4 seconds.

5 Repeat this cycle five times.

Depression

Depression is not just sadness. Every human being has experienced or will experience sadness. This is a normal part of life, and we learn how to adjust to periods of sadness in our lives. The American Psychiatric Association defines "major depressive disorder," also known as depression, as a common and serious medical illness that negatively affects the individual, the way they feel, think and act (APA, 2020).

Depression can range from mild to severe. To remember the symptoms that make up the diagnostic criteria, I use the SIG-E-CAPS mnemonic.

DIAGNOSTIC CRITERIA FOR DEPRESSION

S	**Sleep changes:** insomnia at night and sleepy during the day
I	**Interest in things is decreased:** usual things that were pleasurable before no longer interest
G	**Guilt:** a sense of worthlessness
E	**Energy:** lack of energy and fatigue
C	**Concentration:** poor concentration
A	**Appetite:** most commonly loss of appetite, but can also be increased appetite
P	**Psychomotor:** includes how the person moves, for example, agitated or lethargic
S	**Suicidal thoughts or preoccupation**

Depression is very common among my patients with chronic pain. And chronic pain is very common among people with depression. It is hard to know which came first, the chronic pain or depression. The most important steps are to identify the symptoms as early as possible, seek a proper medical diagnosis and introduce treatment.

TREATING DEPRESSION

There are various effective strategies to treat depression. Depending on the severity, medications and admission to a hospital ward may be necessary. Other interventions include a change in diet, sleep hygiene, physical activity and mental health counseling.

I recommend the 5Ps of treatment for depression: plate, pillow, physical, pills and psychology. It's a helpful reminder to consider all the tools in our toolbox.

WATCH MY VIDEO ON DEPRESSION

What is postpartum depression?

Postpartum depression is a serious condition that requires treatment and emotional support for a new mother. It is depression that lasts longer than 10 days after a woman gives birth to a new child. Do not confuse it with "baby blues," which is normal for new mothers, who may experience a short period of mood symptoms, lasting less than 10 days.

Are menopausal women at risk for depression?

A woman who enters menopause is at higher risk of developing depression due to the hormonal and emotional changes in her body. Menopause means that the ovaries stop producing eggs and there is no more production of estrogen and progesterone. Symptoms of menopause may include insomnia, hot flashes, mood swings and weight gain. This can look like depression, but it is not the same thing. When menopause symptoms are severe and debilitating, a woman may choose to speak to her doctor about hormone replacement therapy.

THE 5PS TO TREAT DEPRESSION

PLATE	The neurotransmitters in your brain are made up from the nutrients that you eat	Dopamine, the pleasure neurotransmitter, is made up from amino acids that we eat. Serotonin, the happiness neurotransmitter, is made up from tryptophan, an essential amino acid.
	Inflammation	An anti-inflammatory diet helps to reduce inflammation in the body, which improves mood. (See anti-inflammatory diet in *Step 4: Fix Your Diet*, page 148.)
	Gut bacteria	The gut microbiome produces substances that regulate mood.
	Eliminate junk food	Cut down on processed food, pop and added sugars.
PILLOW	Sleep problems can lead to depression. Depression can lead to sleep problems.	Improve sleep efficiency by changing some habits. (See *Step 3: Get Quality Sleep*, page 126.)
PHYSICAL EXERCISE	Exercise releases endorphins, the feel-good neurotransmitters, our endogenous opioids.	Try to achieve 150 minutes of exercises every week. Benefits: mood, distraction, confidence, self-esteem, social interaction, build muscles and flexibility
PILLS	Antidepressants	Your doctor may find one that works for you. Options include: • Selective serotonin reuptake inhibitors (SSRIs) • Serotonin norepinephrine reuptake inhibitors (SNRIs) • Tricyclic antidepressants (TCAs) • Monoamine oxidase inhibitors (MAOi) • Other atypical antidepressants
PSYCHOLOGY	Cognitive behavioral therapy (CBT)	You will learn to identify and manage negative thoughts and behaviors patterns that contribute to depression.
	Other mind-body therapies	A variety of other techniques can be used to relax the body and mind.

Substance-use disorder / addiction

Addiction is a mental health disease. It is not a sign of poor character or a weak person. The medical name for this disease is substance-use disorder. It is a disease of the reward system, in which the proper production of the pleasure neurotransmitter dopamine is disturbed.

People can have this disorder with a variety of substances:

- Alcohol-use disorder
- Nicotine-use disorder
- Opioid-use disorder
- Cannabis-use disorder
- Benzodiazepine-use disorder
- Cocaine-use disorder
- Amphetamine-use disorder

YOU'RE NOT AN ADDICT

We avoid using the term "addiction" because it stigmatizes the person who has the disease. Terms such as "addict" or "junkie" should not be used to describe someone who suffers from a disease of the reward system. The proper term is substance-use disorder. It says that the person has a disease, not that the person is a bad human being.

The substance, for example, opioid, will release high levels of dopamine and will activate the receptors in the brain that cause a pleasant sensation. For this reason, the person with substance-use disorder will find very little pleasure in activities such as completing a task, meeting a deadline, enjoying the company of friends and family, eating a nice meal, learning something new or having sex. Their brain is modified and they require higher amounts of dopamine to feel "normal." These high peaks of dopamine are achieved by using external substances.

The person who suffers from a substance-use disorder will have strong withdrawal symptoms, and they will try to do anything to avoid them. They may even resort to criminal activities to obtain the substances that give them temporary relief.

(For more about substance-use disorders, especially as related to opioids, see *Step 6: Check Your Medicine Cabinet*, on page 204.)

It is very difficult to help a patient to conquer chronic pain if they are facing a substance-use disorder. But substance-use disorder is a treatable condition. Conquer your substance-use disorder and you are much closer to conquering your pain.

COMMON SUBSTANCE-USE DISORDERS

Substance-use disorders can occur with prescribed medications, such as opioids, benzodiazepines or barbiturates. It is not uncommon to see people with chronic pain who use some of these medications, and unfortunately many develop a use disorder to one or more of these substances.

- **NICOTINE** has some analgesic properties, but it causes so many other complications that the pain relief is not worthwhile. Smokers have impaired bone healing, low tissue oxygenation, less cardiovascular capacity and risks of blood clots. Smoking is very common among patients with chronic pain; approximately one in three smoke cigarettes regularly. (See page 211 for more about nicotine-containing products.)
- **ALCOHOL** is used by one in four patients with chronic pain to relax and sleep faster. Withdrawal can be very serious and life-threatening.
- **OPIOIDS,** derived from the opium poppy, are the most potent painkillers. They lead to physical dependency very quickly and in some people, they cause euphoria.
- **CANNABIS CONTAINS THC,** which is the cannabinoid that causes euphoria and relaxation. It has some effects on neuropathic pain and has been used by patients with chronic pain. It can cause physical dependence and withdrawal symptoms when stopped.
- **BENZODIAZEPINES** are used to reduce anxiety, treat panic attacks and sedation. People who use benzodiazepines regularly become dependent, and stopping these medications will cause rebound symptoms such as severe insomnia.

> Substance-use disorder is a disease of the reward system.

How do I know if I am drinking socially or if I am becoming an alcoholic?

Canada's low-risk drinking guidelines suggest the maximum is 10 drinks a week for women, with no more than 2 drinks a day most days; and 15 drinks a week for men, with no more than 3 drinks a day most days (CCSA, 2018).

If your doctor wants to assess if you have a problem with alcohol or other substances, they will ask questions related to how your use is affecting your relationships and employment.

BENNY, SURVIVOR OF A MOTORCYCLE COLLISION

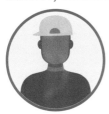 Benny was 19 years old when he had a severe motorcycle accident that caused brain injury, various nerve injuries, fractures and chronic pain. He was in the intensive care unit for many weeks, in rehabilitation for a few months and was discharged home with prescriptions of various opioids, sleeping medications, antidepressants and anti-inflammatories.

Over the months we were able to reduce all his medications and he returned to work. However, when he was 23, he was still using opioids every day. He was concerned he was becoming addicted, as it was getting very difficult for him to live without these pills. Every time he skipped a dose, he felt withdrawal symptoms, including tremors, diarrhea and insomnia. He was getting anxious about not being able to get these pills if the doctor decided to stop prescribing for him. He acknowledged that he used them to "feel normal," and that if he didn't take them, he would feel sad, anxious and tired. He was taking 12 tablets of short-acting oxycodone every day.

He was determined to stop, and I agreed to help him. We started on a tapering plan to gradually reduce the number of pills per day. We planned this would take about 12 to 15 weeks.

A month later Benny came back. He was happy and had stopped completely taking the oxys. He didn't need them anymore.

I was very curious about what he had done. To my surprise, he had downloaded a free app to his cell phone. It was a self-hypnosis app. He said that every time he felt the urge to take an oxy, he would open the app and practice 5 to 15 minutes of self-hypnosis, and the cravings went away.

This for me was a great example of how our mind can control our body. Craving is a very real symptom and it is usually what leads to substance-use disorders.

Can You Have More than One Unhealthy Emotion?

In theory, it is easier to separate and explain these emotions individually, but in practice, they are very hard to distinguish from each other and they usually occur in combination.

In my clinic, I always apply the questionnaires that I have mentioned to detect injustice experiences, fear-avoidance behaviors, generalized anxiety, depression and adverse childhood experiences.

Fear of pain has serious consequences. A person who has high degree of pain-related fear will pay more attention to pain and their pain will interrupt normal daily activities. There is also some evidence that the more attention a person pays to pain, the higher the intensity of pain that the person feels.

> **Pain catastrophizing: always imagining the worst possible scenario**

In addition, I use the Pain Catastrophizing Scale (PCS), a questionnaire created by Sullivan, Bishop and Pivik (1995). The questionnaire has 13 questions in three domains: *helplessness, rumination* and *magnification*.

- "*Catastrophization:* when the person believes that the worst possible scenario will happen, and if it happens, it will be a massive catastrophe"
- "*Helplessness:* a feeling of powerlessness or inability to influence a situation"
- "*Rumination:* a form of thought that persists and is focused on a harmful content, resulting in anxiety and emotional distress"
- "*Magnification:* a type of irrational thought that makes the problem bigger or gives more importance to the situation than it is" (Sullivan, Bishop and Pivik, 1995)

Pain catastrophizing combines worry, anxiety and depression. The term "pain catastrophizing" implies that the pain is more threatening than it is. There is an association between higher levels of pain catastrophizing and more disability from chronic pain. It is fascinating to note that people who tend to catastrophize will report higher pain intensity in various situations, such as a medical procedure or surgery.

Some examples of statements in the PCS questionnaire (1995) are:

- "There is nothing I can do to reduce the intensity of the pain." (helplessness)
- "I keep thinking about how much it hurts." (rumination)
- "I keep thinking of other painful events." (magnification)

> Frida Kahlo, a Mexican artist in the 1940s, portrayed her excruciating pain from a bus accident when she was 17 years of age. She depicted her hopelessness and brokenness in *The Broken Column* and *Without Hope*.

Facing your feelings

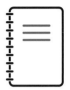

Let's do an exercise. Now that you have learned more about different emotions, what are you going to do about them?

1 Think about how you were feeling in the past, what your feelings are today and what you want them to be in the future.

2 Get your journal and draw faces for what you look like based on how you feel. Then write down your responses.

FACING MY FEELINGS

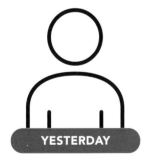
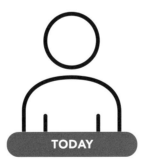
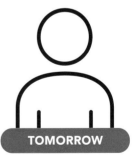

Yesterday, I felt:

_____

Today, I feel:

_____

Tomorrow, I hope to feel:

_____

> What have you learned so far about your emotions? I would love to hear. Share with me on social media using the hashtag #ConquerPain WithDrFurlan.

Mind-Body Therapies

We've already seen some mind-body therapies to help you retrain your brain in the previous chapter. There are many psychotherapy interventions that are helpful to alleviate emotional problems in people with chronic pain. These use many different approaches and strategies. The most effective therapies will include neuroscience education, physical activity, analyses of thoughts and behaviors, stress management and lifestyle modifications.

Cognitive behavioral therapy

The "cognitive" part of cognitive behavioral therapy (CBT) is about what we think and the interpretations that we give to the things we are feeling. Sometimes, what we think about is not correct or helpful.

CASE STUDY

JASPREET AND HIS FIXED BELIEFS

Jaspreet was a 29-year-old male who had a lumbar sprain at work when he carried a heavy box in the office. He came to me having had chronic low back pain for eight months and told me that he could not work because of the pain.

The fact was that he had physically healed and his body was able to do the work, but he was afraid of reinjuring his back. He was afraid his back would deteriorate and he would end up in a wheelchair. His thinking was wrong, and his thoughts were dictating what he could do or not do.

Our interprofessional team provided him with education about pain that helped him understand that what he believed to be true about his pain was not true. They also helped him learn how to problem solve, meditate, relax when he was tense and pace his day-to-day activities. The physiotherapist showed him that he could carry weights safely without damaging his lower back. Now, Jaspreet is back to work!

In the case of Jaspreet, his thoughts were telling him that he could not work, but his thoughts were wrong. While this is an extreme case, I see people with chronic pain all the time who have "wrong thoughts" and need someone to help them to think about what they are thinking. This is the cognitive part of CBT.

The "behavioral" part of CBT is about what you do when you have chronic pain. For example, you can pace your activities instead of overdoing them. When you are thinking differently, you are ready to do things differently and find more enjoyment and less pain in what you do.

CBT is often offered by psychologists or trained mental health counselors. Unfortunately, these can be very expensive therapies. However, more recently, therapists have developed online groups for CBT and computer-based CBT. Many of these are free or very low cost and research indicates that they are effective. I recommend CBT to many of my patients.

MIND-BODY AND PSYCHOLOGICAL THERAPIES FOR CHRONIC PAIN

- ☑ Cognitive therapy and cognitive-behavioral therapy (CBT)
- ☑ Acceptance and commitment therapy (ACT)
- ☑ Mindfulness-based therapy
- ☑ Meditation
- ☑ Relaxation
- ☑ Biofeedback
- ☑ Hypnosis
- ☑ Guided imagery
- ☑ Mirror therapy
- ☑ Pain neuroscience education
- ☑ Somatic tracking

Biofeedback

Biofeedback involves a device or instrument that measures in real time the stress responses of your body, such as hand sweats, heart rate or blood pressure. These measures are presented as a visual representation or auditory sound to you as a marker of their stress at the moment. You then learn techniques to reduce your stress levels and you see or hear the feedback from the machine or device in real time.

I've seen some simple devices and some very sophisticated immersive virtual environments that do this. There are also some apps for smartphones that track your body response to a relaxation or meditation exercise.

It is not only about the relaxation. It is also about shifting your attention and providing an objective and precise understanding of what is going on in both your body and your mind and how they influence each other.

Biofeedback treatment has been shown to be effective for pain in children. It is also used for phantom limb pain, which is a pain associated with a limb that has been amputated. The main problem with biofeedback is that these sessions are usually expensive when done under supervision by a psychotherapist.

Mindfulness

Mindfulness is sometimes referred to as mindful meditation or mindfulness-based stress reduction. (We looked at mindfulness as a way to retrain your brain in the previous chapter.) This kind of therapy is focused on building awareness and accepting of "here and now" experiences, including pain and emotions. You are trained to feel body sensations and emotions in a non-judgmental way.

Meditation training sessions are usually done in group and may involve three components:

- A body scan to pay attention to the entire body, from the tips of your toes to the top of your head, and all the sensations coming from the body
- A sitting meditation usually involving breathing exercises
- Some stretching or posture exercises to finish

The benefits of mindfulness for pain are usually achieved in people who practice meditation every day.

CHANGE ONE LETTER: MOVE FROM MEDICATION TO MEDITATION

I have many patients who were able to reduce the use of opioids just by doing meditation! They tell me that one session of meditation is as effective as taking one tablet of their painkiller. Research from around the world supports the effectiveness of mindfulness-based therapies.

MEDICATION

MEDITATION

Yoga

Yoga is very similar to mindfulness-based therapies. It places emphasis on mental fitness as well as physical fitness. It combines breath control, meditation and exercises to strengthen and stretch the muscles.

Many research studies show that yoga is helpful for people with low back pain, fibromyalgia, arthritis and migraines. It is also a good tool for retraining the pain system. (See page 72 in *Step 1: Retrain Your Pain System.*)

One great advantage is that there are many resources on the Internet teaching yoga and my patients can access them from home. I tell them they need to practice for at least 45 minutes a few times a week to notice the benefits for chronic pain. However, there are so many types of yoga these days, some more vigorous and done in a heated environment. Be careful and ask the instructors if their type of yoga is appropriate for people with chronic pain.

Hypnosis and guided imagery

Hypnosis involves entering an altered state of consciousness through focused attention and helpful "suggestions." The suggestions help you to change our sensations, thoughts and emotions, in other words, "what you feel, what you think and what you want."

Medical research studies have demonstrated that hypnosis helps to reduce the perceptions of pain in our mind. It is also helpful in reducing the unpleasantness of pain and the use of opioids. Studies show that in surgical procedures or acute pain, the perceptions of pain are much reduced with hypnosis.

Earlier in this chapter, I mentioned a young patient who successfully stopped using opioids for chronic pain by using a self-hypnosis app on his phone. I was amazed but not entirely surprised, since the research supports what he told me.

Guided imagery involves active imagination of visual, auditory and body sensations and perceptions. The person imagines doing the movements. Then someone will touch the body part that they are imagining moving and will ask them to focus on the skin sensations and practice the exercises in their head, without moving the body parts. Then the person starts actually doing the movements.

> Hypnosis can help you to change what you feel, what you think and what you want.

Both hypnosis and guided imagery aim at reducing pain by using focused attention and imagination to substitute sensations that are pleasurable on the painful body areas. It seems that these two therapies work better for acute pain conditions but clearly can be helpful for some people with chronic pain.

Acceptance and commitment therapy

I recommend acceptance and commitment therapy (ACT) to many of my patients. Unfortunately, there are not many professionals who are trained to offer ACT. This therapy emphasizes the importance of accepting pain and focusing on goals that are important to the person.

I like it because it is values-oriented and personalized. I see many patients put their lives on hold because of their pain. I feel sorry for them, because they are missing out on important events, such as family reunions, raising their children and achieving their life's goals. Or they have lost jobs or stalled in their careers.

ACT has been transformative for many of my patients. They accept that their pain is here to stay and then they move on with their life goals because they are in control of what they can or cannot do.

How do I know which mind-body therapy is best for me?

It is hard to know which mind-body therapy will work best for each person with chronic pain. It is the same thing with medications: we prescribe a drug to treat pain, but we will only know for sure if the drug is helpful or not after the patient tries it for a while. The same thing with exercises. There are different types of exercises and people have preferences and respond differently to each type of exercise. Some patients like aqua fitness, others prefer jogging, and others will improve by going to a gym and doing weight lifting. When you start a mind-body intervention, it is important to give it time. You need to learn the techniques and practice them regularly. You may not see results immediately. Some people will prefer meditation, others will improve with mindfulness and there are people who need more than one type of mind-body intervention.

I am already doing mind-body therapies and I am still in pain. What should I do?

The first thing to ask is "What is the purpose of this mind-body therapy?" Is it to eliminate the pain or to improve my resilience to pain? These are two different concepts.

If the purpose of the mind-body therapy is to reduce the pain intensity, then this type of therapy is not working for you. You need to find another therapist or try a different mind-body intervention for that purpose.

In case of nociplastic pain, the purpose of the mind-body intervention might be to eliminate the pain completely. That is because the cause of the pain is in the pain system, in the emotions and the mind itself, so treating the mind will fix the pain system and the pain will disappear.

But when the pain is nociceptive or neuropathic, then the purpose of mind-body intervention is not to eliminate the pain but to improve the person who has the pain. We call this improving resilience. In that case, if the person is not noticing any benefit to improve their resilience, they should seek a different therapist or try another type of mind-body intervention.

I remember one patient who finished her ACT sessions and returned for a follow-up visit. She was so different, so much happier. She didn't even talk about her pain with me; she only talked about her life. When I asked her "How is your pain?" she said, "It is still there, but I don't pay attention to it anymore, so it is not bothering me. I have so many other things in life to do. I don't have time to marinate in the misery juice anymore."

ACT is a fairly new treatment, but a growing number of research studies support its effectiveness in helping people with chronic pain to get on with their lives.

"Acceptance and commitment therapy has been transformative for many of my patients."

Medications to Treat the Mind

In *Step 6: Check Your Medicine Cabinet,* we look at a range of medications useful in treating chronic pain. Here, we focus on examples of medications we use to regulate the neurotransmitters in the brain. These are useful in cases where a person has serious unhealthy emotions, such as thoughts of ending their life or harming someone.

ADVANCES IN SCIENCE

The fields of psychiatry, psychology and pain neuroscience have made huge advances in the past century. Previously, we knew little about neurotransmitters and we could not see the brain functioning.

More recently, brain imaging with electroencephalography (EEG), positron emission tomography (PET) scans, functional magnetic resonance images (MRIs) and optogenetics has revealed many functions of the brain, brainstem and spinal cord.

We have a lot more information now about how the brain develops from in-uterus to adolescence and about chemical imbalances, genetic factors, environmental influences and the importance of nutrition and gut bacteria.

The first antidepressant and antipsychotic medications were tested in the early 1950s. Since then, other generations of psychiatric medications have emerged, with better results and less adverse effects.

PSYCHIATRIC MEDICATIONS AND CHRONIC PAIN

Many people with chronic pain have co-existing psychiatric diseases that affect each other. When the pain is well managed, the psychiatric condition is also easier to manage, and vice-versa.

It is important to recognize a psychiatric diagnosis and initiate treatment as early as possible. This can help to avoid worsening of symptoms, isolation, stigma and disability and to prevent deaths.

There are many psychiatric medications used to treat chronic pain — not because they are used to treat a psychiatric co-morbidity, but because their effects are on the pain system and are independent of the psychiatric symptoms. These medications include some antidepressants such as duloxetine and amitriptyline. Other psychiatric medications are used to help patients with chronic pain reduce their depression or anxiety or to sleep better. (For more about using antidepressants to treat chronic pain, see *Step 6: Check Your Medicine Cabinet,* on page 204.)

- **ANTIDEPRESSANTS:** medications to improve mood and depression
- **ANTIPSYCHOTICS:** medications to treat psychosis and schizophrenia
- **ANXIOLYTICS:** medications to reduce anxiety, panic attacks and post-traumatic stress disorders (PTSD)

Trauma-Informed Care for People with Chronic Pain

A history of psychological trauma is very common among patients with chronic pain.

Adverse childhood experiences (ACEs) predispose a child to develop health conditions in adult life, including fibromyalgia, depression and substance-use disorders. (For more about ACEs, see pages 51–53 in *Getting a Diagnosis.*)

Post-traumatic stress disorder (PTSD) is commonly associated with chronic pain, and in some people is what triggers the acute pain to become chronic.

The purpose of trauma-informed care is not to treat symptoms related to the trauma, such as the sexual abuse or assault that happened to that person. Instead, it is meant to provide a supportive environment where people with previous psychological trauma are respected and will not be re-traumatized.

A trauma-informed approach acknowledges that trauma is common. It promotes an environment of healing and recovery, rather than services that may inadvertently re-traumatize. Activities that may re-traumatize the person include having to retell their story, people using labels that stigmatize (such as "addict"), being subjected to procedures that require removing clothes, and punitive or coercive practices.

The five principles of trauma-informed care are safety, choice, collaboration, trustworthiness and empowerment.

"Be kind to yourself, and that includes taking care of your body and mind."

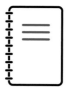

Action plan for unhealthy emotions

Let's do another exercise. Now is a good time to apply what you have learned about your emotions and how they affect your body.

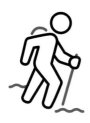

After reading this chapter, you may suspect that you are suffering from fear-avoidance behaviors.

Have a conversation with your doctor or therapist and ask if there are unhealthy emotions that could be delaying your journey to conquer your chronic pain. It might be possible that the answer is no. There are no issues to be concerned about and nothing that you need to do right now.

Or your next step may be to move more and not be afraid that movement will set you back. Your goal may be to increase your daily physical activity levels.

1 Get out your journal and spend some time brainstorming ideas in response to these questions:

- Which unhealthy emotions do you have?
- Who will you talk to about them?
- What are your goals?

2 Write your next steps in bullet points. Maybe you will want to call a mental health counselor, talk to your family doctor or book an appointment with your social worker.

MY ACTION PLAN

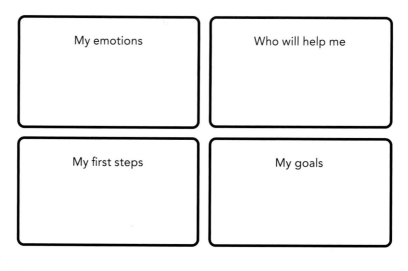

My emotions

Who will help me

My first steps

My goals

CONCLUSION

In this chapter, we looked at some emotions that are unhealthy and how they can interfere with your journey to conquer chronic pain.

KEY POINTS TO REMEMBER

- Your mind is your most potent weapon against chronic pain.
- The mind is where pain is interpreted: it tells us what we feel, what we think, what we remember and what we want.
- Your conscious and unconscious minds give you contradictory messages that can interfere with our feelings about pain.
- Emotions such as sadness and anger are part of the pain experience, not just a consequence from being in pain.
- Fear of pain leads to disability, while confronting the pain and being active leads to recovery.
- Memory of pain is still felt by the brain even after an injury is healed.
- People with chronic pain have higher rates of emotional problems, most commonly, anger, fear, anxiety, depression and substance-use disorder. These are generally an expected reaction of our body, but sometimes they are excessive and need treatment.
- There are many kinds of useful therapies for negative thoughts and emotions.
- You can learn to prevent and to treat these emotional problems.

LOOKING AHEAD

If a person with chronic pain does not have quality sleep, they don't have energy to do what it takes during the day to fight and conquer their pain. In the next chapter, we will look at the relationship between chronic pain and poor sleep and how to improve sleep efficiency without medications.

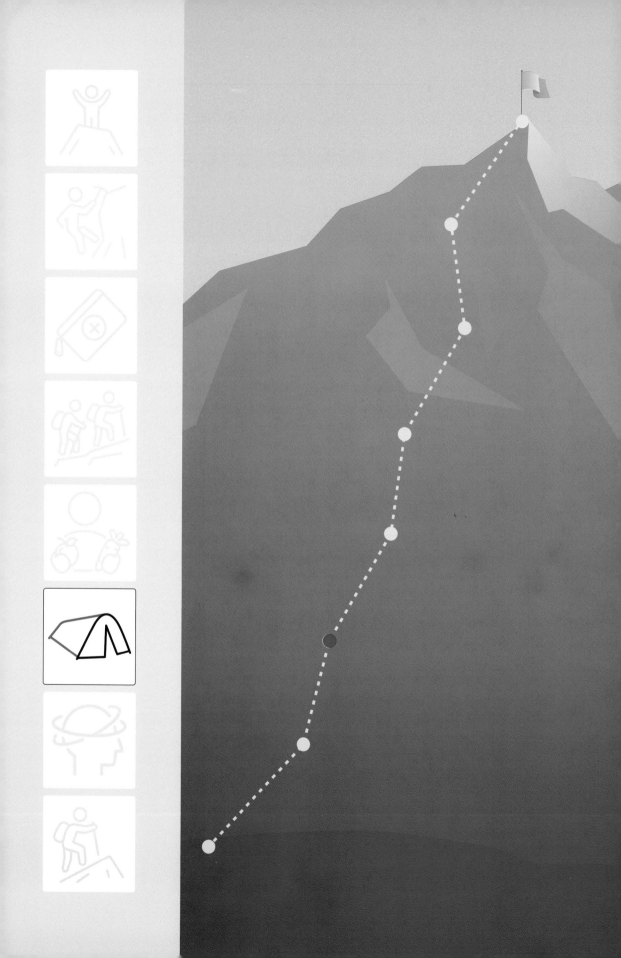

Get Quality Sleep

The aspiring mountaineer needs to adjust their sleep a few weeks before they go to the mountain. They cannot expect to have a perfect first night of sleep in the mountain if their body is not trained to fall asleep quickly, to remain asleep the whole night and wake up refreshed in the morning. This routine requires discipline, and it takes weeks to a few months for the body to develop an efficient sleep cycle. The mountaineer can't risk having insomnia or poor-quality sleep. It could cost their life if they are not alert during the day.

In this chapter we will see how important sleep is to our well-being, especially among people with chronic pain. Most people would agree that chronic pain causes poor sleep, but what many don't know is that poor sleep itself also causes chronic pain. We will also look at the actions you can take ensure you get good, quality sleep and how to improve sleep efficiency without medications. These actions are what we call good sleep hygiene.

Sleep is your energy factory. The better you sleep, the faster your body will heal. Sleep quality is not the same as sleep quantity. Sleeping more is not always the answer. You have to learn and practice to sleep efficiently. This means falling asleep faster, not waking during the night and waking up recharged and ready to face the day.

BIA, THE WOMAN WITH NO NIGHTS AND NO DAYS

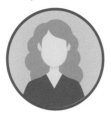 Bia was a 35-year-old interior designer, single, successful and intelligent. She was a passenger in a car that was rear-ended on the highway. She sustained a concussion, neck injury and a fracture of the thigh bone. She had surgery to fix the fracture and attended physiotherapy for many months.

Three years later, when she came to my clinic, she was taking 11 medications daily: various opioids, two antidepressants, antipsychotics, anticonvulsants, various anti-inflammatories and stimulants. Despite all these medications, she still had constant pain in her head, neck and lower back. She had not been able to work since the accident. She had lost her apartment because she couldn't pay the mortgage. She was living in a government-subsidized apartment and receiving a monthly disability payment from the car insurance. She would barely leave her house and she didn't have any friends. She was isolated and lonely.

She had no sleep schedule. She would sleep whenever her body felt tired. She stayed in bed most of the time, watching TV or browsing the Internet. She would fall asleep anytime and sleep as long as she wanted. If she had insomnia, she would take her opioid pills, and if she wanted to stay awake, she would take her stimulants. Sometimes she would go for weeks without opening the curtains, so she would not even know if it was day or night. She would only know when it was daytime if she had medical appointments. Many times she missed her appointments because she was unable to wake up.

She did not get to this point immediately after the accident. It started gradually and she didn't worry about it. She didn't think it was important to maintain a sleep schedule.

Our team worked with Bia for a couple of sessions and we explained the importance of good sleep hygiene. She committed to an action plan. She set SMARTer goals for her sleep routine and made one change at a time. It took her a couple of months to regulate her sleep, but after she conquered that step, we were able to help her with her next phase, which was reviewing and eliminating some of the many medications she was taking.

Chronic Pain Affects Sleep and Poor Sleep Leads to More Pain

Many people with chronic pain ignore the fact that sleep is important to maintain their health. If a person with chronic pain does not have quality sleep, they don't have energy to do what it takes during the day to fight and conquer their pain.

Many people with chronic pain abandon a sleep routine because they are not working, studying or doing regular scheduled activities. They just follow what their body tells them to do.

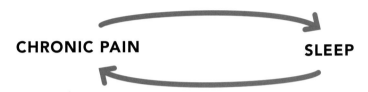

CHRONIC PAIN   **SLEEP**

So, what can we do about this? Here are three points to think about as you begin the work you need to do to recharge your body with quality sleep.

❶ *Achieving a good night's sleep is part of the plan to conquer pain.*

❷ *It is not only your pain that is making you sleep badly.* Most people with chronic pain will say that they don't sleep well because they have pain, and pain wakes them up and interferes with their sleep quality, and that they can't find a good position to sleep because of the pain. That may be true in some cases, but most of the time, the person has developed poor habits, their sleep is superficial and therefore any stimulus will wake them. They perceive that pain is waking them up the whole night, but actually, if they were able to sleep deeper, that pain would not reach their conscious mind and wake them up. Your perception may be misleading you. Most of the time, it is not your pain that is making you sleep badly.

> You need to understand that your perception may be misleading you and, most of the time, it is not your pain that is making you sleep badly.

❸ *You need to stick to a good sleep routine.* Think of this routine as you would training to climb a mountain. You don't have unlimited time to waste. The sooner you get back on track, the easier it will be. The longer you wait to start fixing your sleep, the harder will be on your body. Don't waste another night. Start tonight.

Do You Know Your Sleep Efficiency?

You can calculate your sleep efficiency with some simple math. Divide your total sleep time (TST) by your time in bed (TIB).

Let's illustrate with an example:

Joseph went to bed at 10 pm, was reading until 11 pm, tried to sleep after 11 pm, but wasn't able to fall asleep until midnight. At 3 am he woke up to go the washroom, drank water and came back to bed, but he was not able to sleep again until 4 am. He woke up at 6 am with the alarm clock, but was so tired that he stayed in bed another hour. Finally, he got out of bed at 7 am because he needed to walk the dog.

Let's calculate Joseph's sleep efficiency:

Time in bed (TIB):
10 pm to 7 am = 9 hours = 540 minutes
Time awake:
10 pm to 11 pm = 60 minutes
11 pm to midnight = 60 minutes
3 am to 4 am = 60 minutes
6 am to 7 am = 60 minutes
60 minutes x 4 = 4 hours = 240 minutes
Total sleep time (TST):
9 hours – 4 hours = 5 hours = 300 minutes
Sleep efficiency (SE):
300 (TST) ÷ 540 (TIB) = 0.56
0.56 x 100% = **56%**

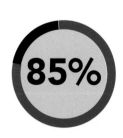

Is 56 percent good or bad? The ideal is above 85 percent.

Higher than 90 percent indicates the person might be sleeping less than their ideal. If you need 9 hours of sleep every night, but you are in bed only 6 hours per night, then it might look like your efficiency is above 90 percent because you fall asleep immediately after going to bed and get up with your alarm clock buzzing on your ear. If that is the case, try to stay longer in bed and see if there are a few minutes before you fall asleep, and if your eyes opened spontaneously before you got up from bed.

Sleep efficiency lower than 85 percent is a problem. This means that you are spending too much time in bed and not sleeping. It could be that you need fewer hours of sleep than you think, or that your sleep is not efficient. In the case of Joseph, he is clearly spending too much time in bed not sleeping. His sleep efficiency is very low. He needs to sleep more or spend less time in bed.

Calculate your own sleep efficiency

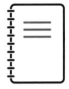

Let's do an exercise. Tonight, before you go to bed, copy the questions below. When you wake up tomorrow morning, answer all of them:

1 What time did you go to bed?

2 What time did you try to sleep?

3 What time did you fall asleep?

4 How many minutes did you stay awake during the night?

5 What time did you wake up?

6 What time did you get out of bed?

If you don't want to do all of the calculations, or you don't remember how many minutes you stayed in bed, there are some apps and fitness trackers that you can use to calculate your sleep efficiency.

Some people will say that everyone needs 8 hours of sleep a night. Well, everyone is different. According to the National Sleep Foundation in the United States, the amount of sleep that adults need is between 7 and 9 hours. We know from scientific studies that less than 6 hours or more than 9 hours is a strong factor in developing chronic pain.

LOWER THAN 85 PERCENT: SLEEP QUALITY NEEDS IMPROVEMENT

If your sleep efficiency is lower than 85 percent, and you don't feel refreshed when you wake up, or you are tired during the day, the solution may not be only increasing the amount of time in bed. It may be that you need to improve the quality of your sleep. There are other conditions that can affect sleep efficiency, such as a sleep disorder, sleep positions or mental health conditions, including depression or anxiety.

> Tell me what you have discovered about your sleep. Did something surprise you? Tag me on social media with #ConquerPainWithDrFurlan.

Ten Tips for Good Sleep Hygiene

There are many scientifically proven methods to improve sleep efficiency and ensure a better quality of sleep. These are the top 10 sleep hygiene tips I recommend to all my patients with chronic pain, especially those who are having issues with sleep efficiency.

1. Get enough light at the right time
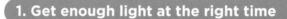

SUNLIGHT IN THE DAYTIME

Try to get exposure to natural sunlight in the morning every day. Natural sunlight or bright white light helps to regulate our brain and tells our brain when it is time to be awake and alert. Have you noticed that you sleep better after you spend a day at the beach?

Go for a walk outside during the day. Open the windows. Move your home office to a well-lit room. If you can't get exposure to sunlight, then make a big light therapy box or buy an artificial white light and turn it on for two hours every morning.

Another advantage of exposure to sunlight is that your brain will produce serotonin, the neurotransmitter of happiness. A lack of sunlight is why some people have seasonal affective disorders (SAD) and feel sad or moody in the winter. They benefit from daily exposure to bright light boxes.

WATCH MY VIDEO ON TEN TIPS FOR IMPROVING SLEEP EFFICIENCY AND SLEEP QUALITY

A study done in 11 nursing homes in Norway used light therapy boxes of 6,000 to 8,000 lux for a period of two hours every day for two weeks. The study showed that older adults improved their sleep efficiency by 80 percent after this regular exposure to bright light (Fetveit and Bjorvatn, 2004).

DARKNESS AT NIGHT

While bright light is good during the day, the opposite is true in the evening. When we are exposed to darkness, our brain will release melatonin, the sleep hormone.

Too much light in the evening or at night is not good, especially blue light, the type of light that is emitted by electronic devices. This includes computers, smartphones, tablets and TVs.

The light in your bedroom is very important. Keep your bedroom very dark when you are sleeping.

A group of researchers from Laval University in Quebec showed that glasses that block blue light prevent the suppression of the sleep hormone melatonin (Sasseville and Hébert, 2010). If you do not wear glasses, the solution is to avoid exposure to blue light in the evening. Banish screens at least two hours before bedtime.

2. Pay attention to what and when you eat and drink

LIMIT CAFFEINE INTAKE

Caffeine is good for waking our brain in the morning because caffeine improves performance and alertness and boosts energy. Avoid any caffeine for at least six hours before bedtime to avoid sleep disruption. Sleep quality is also affected by the amount of caffeine that we ingest in a day. Generally, more than 200 mg of caffeine will affect sleep quality, decreasing total sleep time and prolonging time to fall asleep.

CAFFEINE CONTENT

Coffee = 95 mg caffeine	Green tea = 28 mg
Espresso = 64 mg	Sodas = 22 mg
Black tea = 47 mg	

AVOID ALCOHOL IN THE EVENING

Alcohol blocks the production of melatonin and decreases the production of growth hormones, both of which are important to regulate the sleep cycle.

Alcohol reduces the time the person takes to fall asleep and causes the person to have a deeper sleep in the first half of the night. However, alcohol leads to sleep disruptions in the second half of the night, and total rapid eye movement (REM) sleep is reduced.

REM sleep is the sleep that is important for promoting learning, memory and mood. People who have poor REM sleep have a higher tendency to obesity, type 2 diabetes, migraines and depression.

TRUE OR FALSE?
"Alcohol helps me to sleep better."

This is false!

AVOID HEAVY MEALS BEFORE BEDTIME

Another way to block the production of melatonin and growth hormones is to have a heavy meal right before bedtime, especially a high carbohydrate meal. On the other hand, having a light snack before bedtime helps to improve sleep quality.

3. Avoid drinking liquids before bedtime and getting up at night to pee

If eating a heavy meal is not good at night, the same is true for drinking liquids.

Nocturia is the medical term for getting up at night to pass urine. It may be simply a consequence of drinking too much liquid within two hours before bedtime. If that is your situation, the solution is easy: just stop that habit and remember to empty your bladder before going to bed.

However, nocturia affects 60 percent of older adults and it increases the risks of dying compared to older adults who do not have nocturia. Nocturia can be a sign of a serious disease such as sleep apnea, high blood pressure, diabetes or cardiac disease. In addition, waking up causes sleep loss, a reduction of sleep quality and duration, which then cause more diabetes and obesity. Finally, people with nocturia have a higher risk of falls and fractures, and these injuries could lead to death.

4. Be active and keep moving

There are hundreds of scientific studies showing that regular physical activity improves quality of sleep. In a study of older adults who were sedentary, half of the group was randomized to 16 weeks of moderate-intensity training, while the other half didn't do any exercise. The participants who trained did low-impact aerobics and/or brisk walking for 30 to 40 minutes four times a week. The group that exercised feel asleep faster, slept more, improved their sleep efficiency and felt more rested on awakening than the control group (Hartescu, Morgan and Stevinson, 2015).

Some people prefer to get their exercise during the day, others in the evening. There is conflicting evidence regarding which time of the day is better, so you should find out what works for you. If you do exercise in the evening and have good sleep quality, there is no need to change your routine.

Exercise is more effective at treating insomnia than many medications.

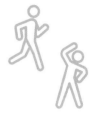

5. Don't take long naps during the day

How common is the siesta? A survey showed that 55 percent of Americans took on average at least one nap during the week, and 35 percent took two or more naps each week. Daytime naps are common in many cultures, especially when the temperatures are higher.

Naps of less than 10 minutes have few if any benefits. Naps of between 10 and 45 minutes have several benefits. Longer naps, however, are associated with loss of performance and sleep inertia.

Sleep inertia is the period of 30 minutes after the person awakens in which there is a low brain speed. This can be very dangerous, especially if the person needs to operate a vehicle or machinery. Sleep inertia is also associated with low performance and low mood that can last for several hours after awakening from a nap.

Which sleep habit did Albert Einstein and Winston Churchill have in common? They were both advocates of a short afternoon nap.

Another problem with longer naps is that it also deteriorates the quality of the night sleep.

In older adults, frequent and longer naps were associated with a 30 percent higher chance of mortality than in individuals of the same age who napped infrequently (Pan et al., 2020). Another study showed that individuals who napped for less than 30 minutes three or more time per week had an 84 percent decrease in the chance of developing Alzheimer's disease (Cai et al., 2021).

You can train your body and mind to take short naps. A short afternoon nap can improve memory and learning. What is the best time to take a nap? Some say it is around 3 p.m.

6. Maintain a regular sleep routine

Practice makes perfect. If you train your body to fall asleep and wake up every day at the same time, you will notice that after a few months you will not need an alarm anymore.

The body follows a circadian rhythm that aligns itself with sunrise and sunset. Having a regular sleep pattern, including on weekends and holidays, can lead to high sleep efficiency and better sleep quality.

7. Reduce the temperature, noise and distractions in the bedroom

Most studies show that a bedroom temperature of around 70°F (20°C) is comfortable for most people. Of course, that also depends on clothing, bedding and personal preferences.

Bedroom noise is very important. Night-time exposure to traffic noise or low-frequency noise affects the levels of cortisol response. Cortisol is the stress hormone, and it peaks in our body around 30 minutes after we wake up. People with poor sleep quality have higher levels of cortisol in the morning. We don't know if higher cortisol leads to poor sleep or if it is poor sleep that leads to higher cortisol.

It is also important to keep distractions out of your bedroom. Use your bedroom only for sex and sleep.

8. Relax your mind and body before bedtime

Mind-body therapies have been shown to improve sleep efficiency and reduce insomnia.

It is impossible to separate the mind from the body.

There are various types of therapies including music, reading a book, mindfulness meditation, prayers, breathing, yoga, visualizations and self-hypnosis.

Some recent preliminary studies showing that binaural auditory beats help to improve sleep and reduce pain (Gkolias et al., 2020). We don't know the exact mechanisms, but it seems they promote connections and neuroplasticity in the brain. Binaural beats occur when two tones of slightly different frequencies are presented separately to the left and right ears. The brain will interpret this as a single tone that varies in amplitude at a frequency equal to the frequency difference between the two tones. This is something like an optical illusion, but it is an auditory illusion. The other names for this phenomenon are brainwave entrainment and frequency following response. If you want to try this, get your stereo headphones and find some binaural music on your phone or the Internet. (Read more about binaural beats in *Step 7: Make Room in Your Toolbox* on page 236.)

> When the mind doesn't relax, the body doesn't relax.

9. Think about natural medicines

Consider taking melatonin and/or magnesium, both natural medicines.

The benefits of **melatonin** are most useful when people are jet-lagged or when they work different shifts. When you need to adjust to a new bedtime routine, melatonin is very helpful in telling your brain that it is time to sleep.

> Take a vacation from melatonin, so it will be effective when you need it.

Studies have shown that 2 mg of prolonged-release melatonin taken before bedtime for three weeks improves the quality of sleep by 34 percent and the person falls asleep nine minutes sooner (Luthringer et al., 2009; Wade et al., 2007). This result is similar to the effects of zolpidem, a prescription medication that shortens the time to fall asleep to about eight minutes.

However, if you take melatonin for three or more weeks, the effects are less noticeable. For that reason, it is not recommended for prolonged periods of time.

Magnesium supplements have a calming effect and improve sleep quality. There are various studies showing that taking magnesium at night helps to improve the quality of sleep and reduce insomnia. Magnesium glycinate has the additional benefit of glycine, which is an amino acid that also has calming effects.

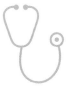

10. Talk to your doctor about your poor quality of sleep

If you practice all of these habits and you still don't have a good quality of sleep, talk to your doctor. A sleep study might be necessary. Certain sleep disorders can affect the quality of sleep and need to be treated. For example, sleep apnea affects 6 percent of Canadians and it is associated with various health problems such as stroke and high blood pressure.

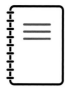

Improve your sleep

Let's do an exercise. Which of these sleep hygiene practices do you need to implement?

- ☑ Get enough light at the right time.
- ☑ Pay attention to what and when you eat and drink.
- ☑ Avoid drinking liquids before bedtime and getting up at night to pee.
- ☑ Be active and keep moving during the day.
- ☑ Don't take long naps during the day.
- ☑ Maintain a regular sleep routine.
- ☑ Reduce the temperature, noise and distractions in the bedroom.
- ☑ Relax your mind and body before bedtime.
- ☑ Think about natural medicines.
- ☑ Talk to your doctor about your poor quality of sleep.

It may be hard for you to change many of your sleep habits at the same time, but make a commitment to change at least one, and then move to the next one on your list.

❶ Try making a priority list. Start with the step that will be easiest for you. Plan how you will achieve your goals. Record your plan in your journal and review regularly to see how you are doing.

I would love to hear your plan to get quality sleep.
Which step was the easiest and which was
the hardest for you to change?
Share with me in social media using the hashtag
#ConquerPainWithDrFurlan.

CONCLUSION

In this chapter, we saw that sleep is very important, especially for people with chronic pain. The 10 strategies to improve your sleep efficiency I have shared here have been proven successful. I recommend them to my patients.

KEY POINTS TO REMEMBER

- Pain can lead to poor sleep, but poor sleep also leads to more pain.
- When you have chronic pain, that doesn't mean you can't get a good sleep. Oftentimes what is causing you to lie awake at night is not your pain but poor sleep habits.
- You can calculate your sleep efficiency by dividing your total sleep time by your time in bed. A good quality sleep is at least 85 percent.
- When the mind doesn't relax, the body doesn't relax. When the body doesn't relax, the mind doesn't relax.
- It is really hard to conquer pain when your sleep is a mess, but fixing your sleep routine can help you climb that mountain.

LOOKING AHEAD

In the next chapter, *Step 4: Fix Your Diet,* we will explore the connections between what we eat and chronic pain and look at how healthy, mindful eating can reduce your pain.

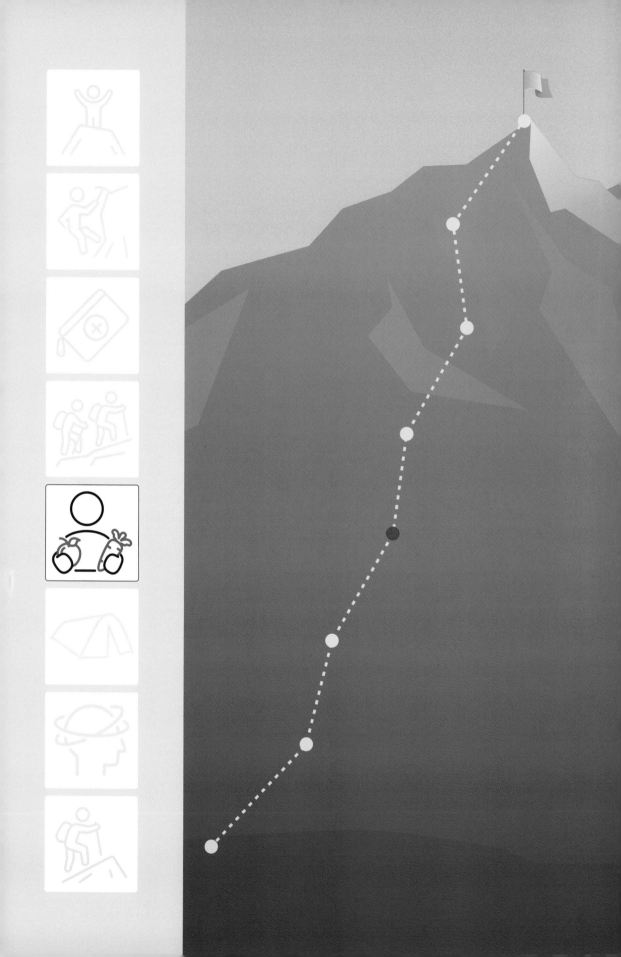

STEP 4

Fix Your Diet

The mountaineers need to bring their food to the top of the mountain. They can't carry heavy loads. They must choose carefully what they eat so they don't lack energy, vitamins, water, proteins and fat. Protein bars are compact sources of healthy nutrients, but they are not always satisfying or pleasurable, so they will also bring some rewarding food that tastes good and that they enjoy. Planning meals is a very important skill and it must be done well in advance of the climbing activity.

In our culture, we eat what is quick, affordable and easy. We eat to comfort our anxiety, disappointments and loneliness. Many people do not understand the connection between their pain and what they eat. This is often a neglected topic in medical practice. Many physicians do not even touch on this aspect of their patient's lives, and it is really a missed opportunity to improve not only their pain, but their mood, sleep, cardiovascular and hormonal health.

In this chapter, we will see why people with chronic pain need to pay particular attention to their nutrition, how choosing nutritious and essential ingredients can help you avoid inflammation in your body and how mindful eating is important. We'll also explore barriers to maintaining a healthy diet and consider vitamins and other dietary supplements.

Nutrition versus Malnutrition

This chapter is not about losing weight, eating your vegetables and drinking more water. I will not bore you with all of that, as I assume you already know that those things are very important.

I'm more concerned if you are malnourished. Yes, malnutrition is not just about children in Africa. According to the US Department of Agriculture, in 2020, one in eight households in the United States had difficulty providing enough food for all its members (USDA, 2022). More than 41 million Americans face hunger, including 13 million children. Causes of malnutrition include inappropriate dietary choices, low income, difficulty obtaining food and various physical and mental health conditions.

CHRONIC PAIN AND NEGLECTING NUTRITION

People with chronic pain tend to neglect their nutrition. The following are some of the explanations that my patients give me:

- "My diet has nothing to do with my pain."

- "My pain is caused by an injury. What I eat or don't eat does not interfere with my pain."

- "I deserve some reward for all the suffering I'm enduring."

- "All of my previous doctors never asked me about my diet, so it must not be important."

- "I can't afford to eat healthy."

- "I tried changing my diet and it didn't make my pain better."

- "I've always been like that, even before I had this pain."

- "Obesity has nothing to do with my pain. I know many obese people who don't have pain."

Do any of these statements sound familiar to you?

"Many people do not understand the connection between their pain and what they eat."

Consider your most recent meal

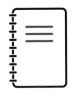

Let's do an exercise. Get your journal. Remember your most recent meal and do a self-assessment by answering these 10 questions:

1 What did you eat? Write down the name of your meal. For example, pasta with tomato sauce; hot dog; soup and salad; pizza, etc.

2 List all the ingredients that are included in that meal. For example, if you had pasta and tomato sauce, did you make the pasta yourself? If yes, then note the type of flour, if you added eggs, salt and so on. Did you prepare the tomato sauce yourself? If yes, then write the type of tomatoes, herbs, garlic, salt, extra virgin olive oil, etc. If you bought the dry pasta and canned tomato sauce, then, copy the ingredients from the packages. If you had a hot dog, you probably did not make the bread or the sausage, so write "I don't know the ingredients."

3 Describe the nutritional values of your meal. Write the total amount of calories, sugars, protein, fat, trans fats, cholesterol, vitamins, minerals and sodium.

4 Record any artificial flavors, sweeteners and preservatives.

5 How long did it take for you to prepare that meal?

6 How long did it take for you to eat that meal?

7 Did you enjoy the aroma, flavor, colors, texture and taste?

8 What was the reason for you eating that meal? For example, you were hungry; you were not hungry yet, but it was your lunch/break time and you had to eat; you were out with friends/family and everyone was eating. Or you didn't have anything else to do; you were craving some comfort food.

9 Was the portion that you ate the right amount, less than you needed or more than you needed?

10 How much did you enjoy the whole experience of eating that meal? Give zero if you disliked it and 10 if it was the most enjoyable meal you ever had.

What my patients eat every day is very important for their health. I take time to ask questions and have a discussion with them about nutrition as a fuel for their body and mind.

I know that not many doctors feel they have expertise in this area and they refer their patients to a nutritionist or dietician. That is acceptable but not ideal.

I am very curious about my patients' overall well-being, including anything that influences their health and could cause diseases. I ask basic screening questions and if I don't see any problems, then we don't need to discuss that anymore. But when I identify some serious red flags in their eating habits, nutrition and diet, then I must intervene. This intervention can be referring them to a specialist dietician or nutritionist or doing something myself.

CONNECTIONS BETWEEN DIETARY INTAKE AND CHRONIC PAIN

- The pain system needs nutrients to work properly. What you eat directly impacts the function of the nervous, immune and endocrine systems and, therefore, your pain experiences.

- Maintaining a healthy weight dramatically reduces pain by reducing the loads on joints and meta-inflammation.

- Chronic pain is harder to manage when there is diabetes, poor mental health or cardiovascular diseases. These are conditions that are directly impacted by dietary intake and weight status.

Nutritional Red Flags

These are the five primary nutritional red flags that I watch for in my patients with chronic pain:

1. Are they using food for the wrong reasons?

2. Are they malnourished?

3. How are they preparing and eating their meals?

4. Do they have a health condition that requires diet modification?

5. Is pain affecting their ability to plan, purchase and prepare their meals?

Before you read the rest of this chapter,
what do you think of these five questions?
Do any of these nutritional red flags apply to you?
Would you like to share with me?
Tag me using this hashtag: #ConquerPainWithDrFurlan

1. Are you using food for the wrong reasons?

EATING WHEN YOU ARE NOT HUNGRY

Sometimes I eat without being hungry. I bring food to my office and I keep eating while working just because I have a deadline or many back-to-back meetings. There are days when I spend hours in front of the computer, especially when every meeting is a videoconference.

Frequently I eat just for the habit, without even noticing what I am eating or without being hungry. The problem is that I overeat or don't pay much attention to what I eat.

If you are not hungry, chances are your body doesn't need more calories. But think about the essential nutrients. Are you getting them? It may be especially hard to get enough of the right vitamins and minerals, because our body is not able to make or store them.

EATING TO RELIEVE ANXIETY

Some people eat to relieve their anxiety. There are many stressors in their lives. Perhaps they need to make a decision or have a challenging conversation with someone. They use food to give them comfort.

Don't we all have our favorite comfort foods? For some, it is chocolate; for others, it is ice cream.

What is the problem with that? The stressor did not go away just because you ate a big bowl of unsaturated fat with 40 g of sugars and artificial flavors. The stressor is still there and you will have to face it. But now, your body has consumed all the calories it needs for 24 hours in one single serving of ice cream.

What will your body do with that ice cream?

1. *Your brain will release dopamine,* the "feel-good" hormone, which will give you immediate pleasure and a sensation of satiety or mission accomplished.

2. *Your pancreas will release a lot of insulin.* An excess of insulin will cause your body to absorb too much sugar, and it can also lead to insulin resistance. The cells in your body become resistant to insulin, increasing your risk of diabetes type 2.

3. *Your body will store all that energy,* just in case you are starving one day and your body has to get energy from somewhere. And the way your body stores energy is transforming everything into fat and storing in the liver, abdomen, hips and everywhere where there are fatty cells.

4. *Your body will tell you to skip the next meal.* Remember that salad you had in the fridge or the fruits you bought? Forget about them; you don't need them anymore. You feel okay now.

5. *You will feel guilty afterward.* Your mind will remind you later that the stressor didn't go away, that you ate what you didn't need, that you didn't eat what you needed, and even worse, you don't even remember the flavor of the ice cream you ate because you consumed it in five seconds. What was it again? Vanilla or chocolate? If you are going to eat ice cream, eat it on a special occasion, and eat mindfully and with moderation.

2. Are you malnourished?

> Being malnourished isn't just about not getting enough food. It can also mean not getting the right food.

According to the World Health Organization, "Malnutrition refers to deficiencies or excesses in nutrient intake, imbalance of essential nutrients or impaired nutrient utilization." Specifically, it includes:

1. Undernutrition, including stunting (low height for age), wasting (low weight for height), underweight (low weight for age)

2. A lack of important vitamins and minerals

3. Overweight, or obesity

4. Diet-related noncommunicable diseases, such as heart disease, stroke, diabetes and cancer

EXAMINE YOUR FOOD BILLS

How would you feel about showing your restaurant and grocery bills to your doctor or nutritionist? If you think that they would approve, you probably are doing the right thing.

> **We are what we eat, and we eat what we buy.**

- Do you frequently eat at fast-food chains? They don't usually cook with the best ingredients and they use a lot of processed meat, added salt and sugars.
- Do you have lots of bills for restaurants or takeout meals? Be careful with the portion sizes, deep-fried stuff, sugary drinks, trans fats and cholesterol.
- Does your grocery bill include a lot of pop, frozen pizza, processed meats, white bread and canned soups? You are probably ingesting much more sodium than you need and unhealthy fats and sugars.

If your buying habits include healthy ingredients to cook your meals at home, this is the first step to a healthy diet. Takeout food and restaurant meals are made to suit the restaurant's owners, not you.

3. How are you preparing and eating your meals?

How you prepare and eat is as important as what you eat. Homemade meals can be much healthier if you know how to cook them. Preparing your meals can be a daunting task for some people, especially if they were raised in a family without these habits. Shopping, preparing and mindful eating are habits generally learned in childhood.

But don't get discouraged if you don't know where to start. Even if you did not learn these skills, it is never too late. There are books, videos and tutorials by people who learned how to take charge of their nutrition.

> Eat healthy, nutritional meals so your body will not let you down when you need it.
>
> Nutrition provides the basis for your brain to develop, for your muscles and bones to sustain you and for your internal organs to work quietly without needing maintenance. It is like your car. If you mix water with the gasoline, or if you don't change the oil, the car will break and let you down.

> ## *"Any money that you save at the grocery store, you will spend later on medicine."*
> — Lourdes, my mom

Cooking at home does not need to be complicated. It requires some planning, organization and discipline, but the time you invest in your nutrition is time you will save going to doctors and hospitals in the future.

PAY ATTENTION TO HOW YOU EAT

In addition to shopping and preparing meals, how you eat is also important. Do you eat mindfully? Do you take time to appreciate your meals? Use your senses to see, smell, taste and touch your food. Take time to eat; do not rush. Avoid distracting electronics such as cellphones, tablets, TV or radio when eating.

If you have family, relatives or friends, eat together to make mealtimes a time for socialization and conversation. If you have small kids around, make every day an opportunity to teach them good healthy habits.

And don't forget to give thanks for what you are eating. Thanks for the hands that planted, raised and harvested the ingredients you eat. Thanks for the earth and rain that nourished the plants and animals in the fields. Thanks for the people who transported the ingredients from one place to another so you can have them at your table. And thanks for the people who prepared your meal for you.

4. Do you have a health condition that requires diet modification?

People with chronic pain may have other health conditions that affect their health. When these conditions are not well controlled, they may aggravate the pain intensity.

> Did you know that the fat tissue in our body produces adipokines? There are more than 100 types of adipokines, and many of them are pro-inflammatory. They cause a chronic, slow, low-grade inflammation that is implicated in causing osteoarthritis, diabetes type II and cardiovascular problems.

These are examples of health conditions that aggravate pain:

Diabetes $\longrightarrow$ **leads to neuropathies** $\longrightarrow$ **nerve damage** $\longrightarrow$ **neuropathic pain**

High blood pressure $\longrightarrow$ **vascular problems** $\longrightarrow$ **poor circulation** $\longrightarrow$ **poor oxygenation** $\longrightarrow$ **nociceptive and neuropathic pain**

Obesity $\longrightarrow$ **fat tissue produces adipokines** $\longrightarrow$ **constant pro-inflammatory state** $\longrightarrow$ **accelerates osteoarthritis** $\longrightarrow$ **nociceptive pain**

I have had patients who tell me, "I don't want to talk about my weight or my diet. I'm here to talk about my pain."

It may not be what they want to hear, but my answer is simple: "Imagine that tomorrow you attached weights to your arms, legs and abdomen, 20 pounds (9 kg) in all. Then imagine doing all your daily activities as usual, but carrying that excess weight the whole day. And not only that, now, for each 10 pounds, you are going to take a tablespoon of adipokines per day, which are pro-inflammatory substances. I expect that you would find that excess weight has increased your pain and make you more tired. Do you agree?"

Usually, they will agree. Carrying excess weight can keep us from feeling our best.

5. Is pain affecting your ability to plan, purchase and prepare your meals?

Unfortunately, chronic pain can be very debilitating. It can affect how a person can plan, purchase and prepare their meals. Pain reduces their ability to plan ahead, shop for food, cook and feed themselves.

It is important to identify situations where this is the reason for nutritional deficiency or inadequate diets. If you feel overwhelmed by the thought of meal planning and preparation, there are professional and volunteer organizations that can help you plan, shop and prepare meals and even come to your home to help you to eat adequately.

"Unfortunately, chronic pain can be very debilitating. It can affect how a person can plan, purchase and prepare their meals."

REASONS WHY PAIN MIGHT AFFECT A PERSON'S ABILITY TO EAT NUTRITIOUSLY

- *Mood disorders* such as depression and anxiety may impair a person's ability to take care of themselves. Because mood disorders are influenced by diet, it is important to eat nutritiously.
- *Sleep disorders* also influence a person's ability to plan, purchase and prepare their meals. People with chronic pain are usually fatigued during the day and sleepless during the night. Tired people make poor choices.
- *Using food and drink to ease pain.* Some people use food and alcohol as aids to sleep, and will indulge themselves, creating other health problems. Caffeine consumption can be high in some people with chronic pain, and adding a treat alongside can mask their hunger.
- *Medications.* Many patients take too many medications that can upset their stomach or cause nausea or constipation. They tend to avoid eating to decrease these symptoms. A common side effect of pain medications is dry mouth, which makes it harder to chew protein or fiber-rich food.
- *Eating is painful.* In some cases, people say they are hurting too much and it is too painful to eat. This is more common in people with TMJ dysfunction, headaches and trigeminal neuralgia.
- *Priorities.* Some people say that dealing with pain can be a higher priority than eating. I had a patient who had to make a choice between getting ready in the morning to go to work or eating breakfast. She said she could not do both as they would take too long.
- *Muscle loss.* Muscles are made from proteins. A poor dietary intake can cause muscle loss. Muscle mass is important for maintaining balance, independence, strength and flexibility and for preventing osteoporosis.
- *Financial restrictions.* Many people with chronic pain have lost their jobs and are on income replacement, disability or workers' compensation or have taken early retirement. Eating healthy can be expensive and eating poorly is much more affordable.
- *Faulty hunger signals.* Many patients tell me that they don't feel hungry when they are in pain. They say that pain overrides their hunger signals. They don't feel like eating.

BEWARE EXPENSIVE "MIRACLES"! EAT HEALTHIER INSTEAD

A lot of advertising and false messaging is aimed at people with chronic pain. Every day a new miracle diet promises to remove all their pain and suffering. These diets tend to be deceiving, expensive and take their focus away from other strategies that are simpler and healthier.

Sometimes my patients will list all the supplements and vitamins they take, but tell me they can't afford to eat healthy. Fast food, restaurants and takeout meals are very convenient. They may give the appearance of healthy food and they seem to be less expensive.

But if you stop to calculate all the unhealthy ingredients you are consuming, the healthy nutrients your body is missing and the money you are spending, it can be eye-opening.

METABOLIC SYNDROME

The American Heart Association (2021) defines metabolic syndrome as a group of five conditions that lead to heart disease, diabetes and stroke. It is diagnosed when the person has three of the five conditions below:

- High blood sugars

- Low levels of the good cholesterol (HDL)

- High levels of triglycerides in their blood

- Large waist circumference, or an "apple-shaped" body

- High blood pressure

A person with metabolic syndrome can reduce their risks of developing a severe consequence by losing weight, increasing physical activity and eating a heart-healthy diet rich in whole grains, fruits, vegetables and fish. These ingredients are also what is recommended in an anti-inflammatory diet.

"Tired people make poor choices."

LUI, THE CHEF WHO ATE JUNK FOOD

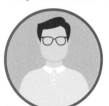 Lui was a chef who immigrated from Korea to Canada when he was 25. He was 30 years old when he came to my clinic at the beginning of the COVID-19 pandemic. He reported that he had had low back pain for many years.

Lui was obese and, even as a teenager, smoked cigarettes and drank a lot of alcohol. He was working at a fast-food chain about 11 hours a day, six days a week. His meals consisted of two large portions a day that he bought at the food court where he worked. He never felt like cooking at home, as he wanted to stay away from a kitchen during his free time. He was 100 pounds (50 kg) above his ideal weight. His cholesterol increased, his blood sugars were always on the upper boundary and his blood pressure was going up. He didn't have time to exercise.

When the pandemic hit, the restaurant closed, and he was sent home for many months. I didn't recognize him when he came for a follow-up appointment six months later. He had lost all the excess weight, he had built more muscle, his skin was tanned, and his blood tests and blood pressure were normal.

He still had lower back pain, but only occasionally. He was not taking any pain medication anymore, and he said he could manage his pain much better. He was able to walk more than 3 miles (5 km) a day and cook his own meals at home. He had quit smoking and was no longer drinking alcohol daily. He wasn't buying junk food or takeout meals. He was eating a very well-balanced menu that included fruits, vegetables, dairy, protein and cereals.

He was very proud of himself, and more confident in his abilities to tackle pain itself. He had more energy and was sleeping better. He was confident that when he would return to his previous routine and job, he would maintain healthier habits. He felt empowered to continue doing what was best for him.

I discharged Lui from my pain clinic, as he had learned how to take care of himself. His chronic low back pain improved dramatically. He still has occasional pain, but his mind and body are prepared to tackle the challenge.

What Is Inflammation?

To understand why an anti-inflammatory diet is so important, first you need to understand what inflammation is.

Inflammation is a normal reaction of the body to any threat, insult, trauma, attack or infection. When there is an injury or a disease, the body will recruit red blood cells to heal the injury or fight the disease. Your immune system reacts by sending white blood cells to combat the insult, for example, to kill the bacteria or eliminate the cancer cells. The immune system always sends a lot of cells because it is safer to err by sending more than risk sending not enough cells. This is what happens in acute inflammation.

THE INFLAMMATORY PROCESS

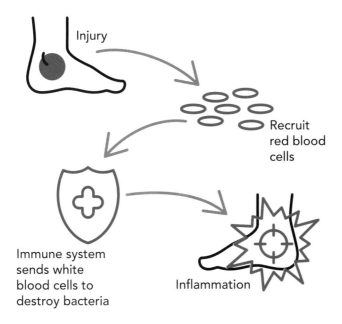

Injury

Recruit red blood cells

Immune system sends white blood cells to destroy bacteria

Inflammation

Acute inflammation always has these four signs: redness, swelling, heat and pain. With situations of chronic inflammation, such as osteoarthritis, these signs may not be visible to the eyes, but they happen microscopically.

Fat tissue releases pro-inflammatory substances called adipokines, such as leptin and cytokines. So even if you stick to an anti-inflammatory diet, your levels of inflammation may not go down because the fat tissue in your body is constantly releasing these pro-inflammatory substances from the excess fat that you are carrying around.

Autoimmune diseases occur when your immune system recognizes your own cells as something that is threatening and then attacks the normal cells. An example is lupus disease, where the immune system attacks the joints, skin, kidneys, brain, heart and lungs.

FAQ

Is fibromyalgia an autoimmune disease?

....

We don't know if fibromyalgia, a chronic pain condition, is an autoimmune disease. However, we have seen that people with fibromyalgia have chronic inflammation going on, because there are some inflammatory markers that are higher in people with fibromyalgia. We don't know if the inflammation is cause or consequence.

An anti-inflammatory diet

An anti-inflammatory diet is a common-sense diet. Here are the main elements:

- *Avoid white bread, white flour and gluten.* Replace with gluten-free flours such as almond flour, oat flour, brown rice flour, corn flour, tapioca or cassava flour.
- *Avoid white sugar, any kind of sugar and artificial sweeteners.* Instead, enjoy homemade sugar-free jams or just plain fruit that already contains sugars.

NATURALLY SWEET
It takes time to retrain your tastebuds to sense natural sugars in fruits, vegetables and milk. Once you train your tastebuds without any added sugar or sweetener you will be surprised how awful it tastes when you add anything to sweeten your drinks or food.

- *Avoid soda, pops and any kind of carbonated drinks.* Replace with water, homemade teas and freshly squeezed citrus oranges, lemons and limes. Or try berry smoothies.
- *Avoid processed foods.* Replace with fresh, raw vegetables and fruits. Instead of processed meat, buy raw meat, poultry or fish, and cook it yourself at home.

PROCESSED FOOD

I find that very few people understand what processed food is. Look at the package of food that you have in front of you. Is it in the original state that you would find in nature?

If it has been cooked, canned, frozen, packaged or changed with fortifying substances or preservatives, it is processed food. For example, fish is very healthy, but if you buy a box where the fish has been prepared in a factory, fried in unhealthy oil, and had preservatives added to last longer in the shelves, it is processed fish.

- *Avoid unhealthy fats* such as trans fats and hydrogenated oils. Read the labels and you will find these unhealthy fats in margarine, shortening, packaged meats, hot dogs, cookies, muffins, cupcakes, frozen pizza, microwave popcorn and more. Replace with healthy fats, such as extra virgin olive oil, canola oil and nuts. Make sure your diet includes polyunsaturated fatty acids (PUFAs) such as omega-3 and omega-6 (see page 153).

> Prepare containers with healthy snacks so they are ready to grab. Individual portions of nuts or fruits are good choices.

- *Reduce red meat.* There is no need to eliminate all red meat from your diet when following an anti-inflammatory diet. (See page 151 about vitamin B_{12} deficiency, which can occur in people who restrict red meats from their diet.) Still, it is good to limit red meat to one or two meals per week. Replace with beans, lentils, chickpeas and whole grains, including kernels, quinoa, bulgur, brown rice and oatmeal. Also highly recommended are green-leaf vegetables such as spinach, kale and broccoli.

> Leafy greens such as spinach, kale and collards are excellent anti-inflammatory ingredients. Keep leafy greens in your fridge clean and ready to eat; toss with olive oil and vinegar and enjoy a big salad. Add them to smoothies, meat or bean dishes.

- *Limit alcohol.* There is no need to eliminate alcohol completely, but there are reasons to reduce: to avoid intoxication, alcohol use disorder and obesity. Alcohol contains a lot of calories. Replace sweetened cocktails, beer and spirits with red wine. One glass of red wine a day is safe and it is rich in antioxidants.

- *Limit coffee.* There is no need to eliminate coffee, as there are benefits, but drinking too much is not healthy. Also, you may be adding too much cream, milk, sugars or sweetener to your diet. Replace some of your coffee with green tea. Green tea contains antioxidants and many healthy compounds.
- *Avoid packaged snacks*, especially when you are in a rush, hungry and tired. You know when you get home, after a long day, and you want to grab a quick bite, sit and relax for a while. That is the dangerous hour. Have some containers with healthy snacks ready to grab.

The anti-inflammatory diet is a healthy diet. Even people who do not have chronic inflammation or chronic pain may benefit from adopting this diet. Of course, your diet is your choice, but I want you to make informed choices that will maximize your well-being and overall health.

My approach is to incorporate healthy eating habits in your life for good. If these changes are overwhelming, try changing one thing at a time. It is better to go slowly and stick to it than to abandon it because you could not persevere.

Vitamins and Other Dietary Supplements

The following vitamins and other dietary supplements are relevant to people with chronic pain. Consult with your doctor or your dietitian to learn which ones may be helpful to you.

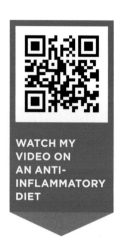

WATCH MY VIDEO ON AN ANTI-INFLAMMATORY DIET

PRO TIP

More is not always better. We need to be careful with supplements and vitamins; they may be necessary, but not in excess.

Vitamin D

Vitamin D helps us to absorb the calcium that we eat in our diet. Calcium is important for bone health. A lack of calcium in the bones is a sign that a person has osteopenia; when the bones are severely deficient, then it is osteoporosis.

Osteoporosis predisposes a person to have bone fractures. These are called fragility fractures because they occur in bones that are usually considered very strong, such as the femur, vertebrae, shoulder and wrists.

Vitamin D is also key to maintaining muscle strength, therefore reducing falls and muscle pain. It is also important to the immune system to fight cancer and infections, and it helps to regulate mood.

OSTEOPOROSIS IS THE SILENT THIEF THAT STEALS CALCIUM FROM OUR BONES

Osteoporosis is silent because it does not have any symptoms and it is impossible to know if you have it unless we do X-rays. There is a special kind of X-ray called bone densitometry that measures how much calcium there is in certain parts of the body and compares it to the normal population.

Our body transforms cholesterol to vitamin D when our skin is exposed to ultraviolet B sunlight. Vitamin D is also found naturally in some foods, such as fish (salmon, sardines, herring, mackerel, trout and tuna), cod liver and egg yolk. In North America, many foods are fortified with vitamin D, including margarine, infant formula, cow's milk, egg products and meal replacements.

If a person is deficient in vitamin D, either because they are not exposed to sunlight or their diet does not contain enough vitamin D, it is recommended they take a daily supplement between 400 and 2,000 international units (IU). If they take higher doses, we monitor the blood levels of 25-OH-vitamin D because it can accumulate and reach toxic levels.

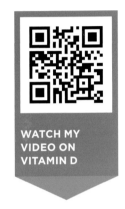

WATCH MY VIDEO ON VITAMIN D

Vitamin K

Vitamin K is essential to the formation of blood clots, which are important to stop bleeding. Without blood clots we could die of hemorrhage. Vitamin K also plays a role in maintaining calcium in our bones, thus preventing osteoporosis and fragility fractures.

It is very easy to obtain vitamin K from your diet. It can be found in green leafy vegetables, sausages, cheese and egg yolk. In some situations, a person has a malabsorption disease (they cannot absorb vitamins from the bowels), such as liver, gallbladder or biliary disease, celiac disease and cystic fibrosis.

Taking supplements of vitamin K does not seem to have adverse effects, but you should check with your doctor because it interferes with blood clots and medications that are used as blood thinners. Vitamin K taken with vitamin D is good for bone health.

WATCH MY VIDEO ON VITAMIN K

Vitamin B$_{12}$

Vitamin B$_{12}$ is essential to forming red blood cells, to neurological function and regulating the synthesis of DNA.

WATCH MY
VIDEO ON
VITAMIN B$_{12}$

Vitamin B$_{12}$ deficiency can be corrected by a diet rich in fish, meat, poultry, eggs, milk and milk products. However, the damage that the deficiency causes in the neurological system is sometimes irreversible. That damage includes pain. For that reason, when a person has vitamin B$_{12}$ deficiency, we still recommend supplementation so the disease will not get worse.

There is some new evidence suggesting that vitamin B$_{12}$ can be used in the treatment of neuropathic pain and low back pain, but more studies are needed to demonstrate these benefits.

Magnesium

Magnesium plays some important roles in people with chronic pain. It blocks a receptor in neurons (NMDA receptor) that transmits pain to the brain; it is a muscle relaxant; and it leads to soft stools, which may help with constipation.

The effect of magnesium in the NMDA receptor interrupts the pain synapses, which helps to avoid central sensitization (nociplastic pain), prevent migraine and treat neuropathic pain.

People with chronic pain may have constipation because they use opioids, because they have a diet low in fiber and water and/or because they don't exercise much. So, constipation can become a real problem, and magnesium is a natural way to restore bowel movements.

WATCH MY
VIDEO ON
MAGNESIUM

Magnesium can be found in a variety of nutrients, including nuts, green leafy vegetables, cereal, potato, beans and many fruits. People do not need to supplement magnesium if they ingest a healthy variety of food.

In case supplementation is necessary, there are many different forms of magnesium. Speak to your doctor, pharmacist or dietitian about which is best for you.

- In **magnesium hydroxide**, or milk of magnesia, the magnesium is not well absorbed, so it stays in the gut and cause soft stools and diarrhea. It is good for constipation.
- **Magnesium citrate** is a form of magnesium bound to citric acid that has a mild laxative effect. This form is one of the forms that is better absorbed. It functions best on an empty stomach followed by a full glass of water or juice to aid absorption.
- **Magnesium glycinate** is a form of magnesium combined with the amino acid glycine, which improves its absorption. Due to the presence of glycine, this form also has a calming effect on your brain and has been reported to improve sleep quality.

Omega-3 and omega-6 polyunsaturated essential fatty acids

Omega-3 and omega-6 fatty acids are called essential fatty acids because they are essential to our nutrition. However, we don't produce them on our own; we must obtain them from our diet.

Cold water fatty fish and seafood are rich in both omega-3 and omega-6. Plant oils and vegetables also contain omega-3, including flaxseed, chia seeds, soybean, canola, walnuts and dark green vegetables such as kale and broccoli. Omega-6 is also found in meat, poultry, eggs, soybeans, corn, sunflower oils, nuts and seeds.

WATCH MY VIDEO ON OMEGA-3

OMEGA-3 FATTY ACIDS ARE ANTI-INFLAMMATORY, WHILE OMEGA-6 ARE PRO-INFLAMMATORY

We do need to have some inflammation in our body; otherwise, we cannot fight viral, bacterial or fungal infections, or kill cancer cells that develop and grow in our body every day.

OMEGA-6
Pro-inflammatory

OMEGA-3
Anti-inflammatory

In North America people eat much more omega-6 in their diet than omega-3. The proportion is 25:1.

In people with inflammatory diseases such as rheumatoid arthritis, the goal is 1:1. In healthy adults, a good goal is 4:1. Remember, the goal is not to eliminate omega-6 fatty acids from our diet; we need them too. The goal should be to increase the amount of omega-3 to maintain a healthy balance.

BENEFITS OF DIET RICH IN OMEGA-3

For people with chronic pain, here are some benefits of a diet rich in omega-3:

- Reduced need to use non-steroidal anti-inflammatory drugs (NSAIDs) such as ibuprofen or naproxen
- Less post-operatory pain levels
- Improved symptoms in painful diabetic neuropathy
- Reduced use of antidepressants
- Fewer symptoms in people with rheumatoid arthritis
- Less painful menstrual cramps, especially when taken with vitamin E
- Better function in people with knee osteoarthritis
- Improved symptoms of inflammatory bowel disease

Osteoarthritis

Osteoarthritis is a chronic, slow-progressing, insidious disease of the cartilage that covers the bone surfaces.

We have cartilage in most of the joints of our body, including the knees, hips, shoulders, elbows, fingers, temporomandibular joint and even in the spine. When osteoarthritis starts, it destroys the cartilage and causes pain, stiffness and deformity. When osteoarthritis affects the spine, we call it spondylosis. Osteoarthritis is a progressive disease caused by slow and microscopic inflammation.

We know that the cartilage is nurtured by the synovial fluid that is produced by the joint capsule. And if we move that joint, more synovial fluid is produced, thereby bringing more natural nutrition to the cartilage. Also, if we have too much fat in our body producing adipokines, which are pro-inflammatory, then the osteoarthritis continues.

The likelihood of your having osteoarthritis is mostly determined by your genetics, so if you have family members with osteoarthritis, your chances are higher to develop this disease. But there are other factors that accelerate the process, including obesity, smoking, trauma to the joint and other joint diseases such as rheumatoid arthritis.

There are a few things that we can do to slow the progression of osteoarthritis. These include regular low-impact physical activity, weight loss and adequate nutrition with an anti-inflammatory diet. (See *Step 7: Make Room in Your Toolbox*, to read more about how movement is an excellent therapeutic intervention to treat chronic pain and fix the pain system. Motion is lotion.)

> Any treatment of osteoarthritis should be implemented only if there are symptoms that are affecting your ability to function, and not because there is a radiological study showing deformities or cartilage destruction.

Glucosamine and chondroitin for osteoarthritis

Scientists have been trying to find a medication that will stop the progression of osteoarthritis. We know that anti-inflammatories are effective to reduce the pain from osteoarthritis. These are medications such as ibuprofen, diclofenac, cetoprofen and celecoxib. But we also know that anti-inflammatories have side effects, such as gastrointestinal bleeding, and they are contraindicated in people who have heart disease, high blood pressure or kidney insufficiency.

Scientists discovered that there is a substance in the joint, called glucosamine, that is important to maintain a healthy

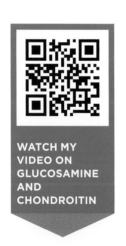

WATCH MY VIDEO ON GLUCOSAMINE AND CHONDROITIN

cartilage. There is another substance called chondroitin that is a component of the cartilage. Once the destruction of the cartilage starts, it is very hard for the body to heal itself and make new cartilage. There are other factors that are important to maintain healthy cartilage, like the deformity of the bones, the weight that the bones have to carry and the amount of movement and exercise that the joint has to do.

Talk to your doctor or pharmacist before you start taking these supplements. If you decide to take glucosamine and chondroitin, here are some things to consider:

- Both glucosamine and chondroitin are relatively very safe, which means they don't cause serious adverse effects like non-steroidal anti-inflammatories or opioids do.
- However, glucosamine and chondroitin can interact with blood thinners like warfarin or coumadin; they can also affect blood sugars, and there is some suggestion that they may increase eye pressure, which could increase the risk of glaucoma.

PRO TIP

Taking glucosamine and chondroitin is not a good replacement for exercising, losing weight and avoiding junk food. If you want to slow the progression of osteoarthritis, choose low-impact physical activity, weight loss and adequate nutrition with an anti-inflammatory diet.

How much glucosamine and chondroitin do you need to take to feel the benefits? And for how long?

It takes weeks or months for the benefits of the glucosamine and chondroitin to be noticed. It is not like a painkiller that you take now and start feeling better in a few hours. You need to take 1,500 mg of glucosamine per day and 1,200 mg of chondroitin per day. The studies that showed beneficial effects for pain recommended for around six months and taking them together. However, other studies showed no real difference compared to a placebo. The results of various studies are conflicting.

How will you know if they work for you or not?

You need to do a before-and-after trial on yourself. Record how much pain you felt and how it affected your function before starting these supplements, and then note how much they improved after six months of taking them.

WATCH MY VIDEO ON COQ10

Coenzyme Q10 for migraines and muscle pain

Coenzyme Q10, or ubiquinone, is a vitamin-like substance involved in providing energy for all the cells in the human body. Our body produces our own CoQ10, and it is present in small, but adequate amounts in our everyday diet. Natural sources of CoQ10 are cold-water fish, meats, vegetable oils, whole grains and some fruits, such as avocado.

Migraines and muscle pain caused by cholesterol-lowering drugs benefit from CoQ10 supplements.

Commit to improving your diet

Let's do an exercise. Get out your journal.

❶ If you identified one aspect of your diet that you can improve, make a commitment to yourself and write it in your journal.

❷ Make your goal a SMARTer goal: specific, measurable, attainable, relevant, time-bound, evaluable and revisable. (We discuss SMARTer goals in *Step 8: Focus on Your Goals*.) Here are some examples:

- I will stop adding white sugar or sweetener to my coffee/tea/juice. Then, I will stop buying white sugar or sweetener.
- I will start cooking a home-made nutritious meal once a week, for one month. Then, I will increase to twice a week, then three to five times a week. After that, I will only eat out or takeout food once a week.
- I will cook fish twice a week and I'll use 4 cups (1 L) of extra virgin olive oil per month. (One person needs approximately 2 tsp (10 mL) per day, so a household of three would use approximately 4 cups (1 L) per month.)

❸ Write your own SMARTer goals. Commit to change one thing at a time. Be patient with yourself; don't expect quick results.

Now that you have read this chapter, did you learn anything new about diet, vitamins and supplements? What did you learn that was new to you? I would love to hear what you think. Tag me on social media using this hashtag: #ConquerPainWithDrFurlan

CONCLUSION

In this chapter, we looked at the connections between pain and what we eat.

Among other subjects, we discussed what malnutrition means. Perhaps you are wondering if you are lacking some essential nutrients. If so, then talk to your doctor or ask to see a nutritionist or dietitian for a thorough evaluation of your nutritional status.

KEY POINTS TO REMEMBER

- Your diet is connected to chronic pain in three ways:
  - The pain system needs nutrients to work properly.
  - Maintaining a healthy weight reduces pain.
  - Chronic pain is harder to manage when there is diabetes, poor mental health or cardiovascular diseases.
- There are many psychological aspects of eating. Using food for emotional reasons may lead to obesity and eating the wrong types of foods — and it does not remove the psychological problem.
- The anti-inflammatory diet is a very good choice for people with chronic pain.
- Consider the various vitamins, minerals and other supplements you may want to take.

LOOKING AHEAD

In the next chapter, *Step 5: Get Help from Others,* we will see how conquering chronic pain is a team effort. We look at how to communicate about your pain with others, including your doctor, partner, family, friends and coworkers. We also touch on the many resources that are available to people with chronic pain, such as pain clinics and peer-support groups.

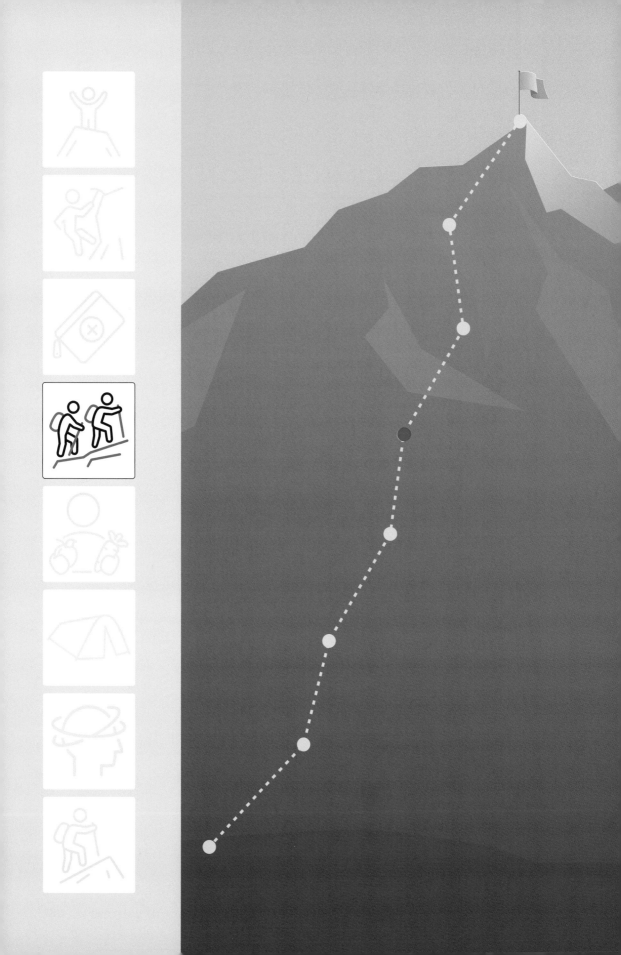

STEP 5

Get Help from Others

Like a mountaineer, you can't get to the top of the mountain all on your own. When preparing for an expedition, a climber will likely hire a coach, join a club or team up with a group. They will need support from close family, coworkers and friends. Those supporters need to know that the person will be on a long expedition and needs time to prepare, to climb and to recover after the challenge. There are solo climbers, but usually a mountaineer does not climb alone. They know it is too dangerous. They also need to have emergency crew aware they are climbing in case they need an emergency rescue. Having a support team will keep the mountaineer feeling safe and focused on their goal as they journey.

Conquering pain involves physical, mental, emotional and social aspects. We call this the bio-psycho-social-spiritual model of pain. The social aspect involves your family, friends, doctors, support groups and the community at large.

In this chapter, we'll see how others can help you in your journey. We'll look at ways to effectively communicate about pain, needs and feelings with family members, healthcare professionals, coworkers and managers, and what to expect from these interactions.

Pain Is Not Just a Biological Phenomenon

By now, you have probably figured out that there is a large emotional component to pain. We know that our emotions have much to do how we perceive pain. If we are happy. we feel less pain; if we are sad, we feel more pain. If we are successful at something, we feel less pain; if we are frustrated and deceived, we feel more pain.

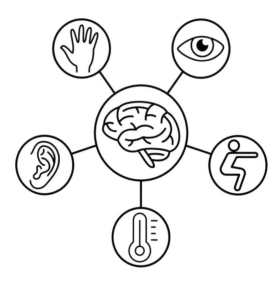

Interpersonal synchronization is a phenomenon that is observed with brain wave patterns where two people get in synchrony. It explains why holding hands with a loved one can sometimes lessen your pain.

The human brain is capable of reducing pain by combining information from past memories, judgment and other sensations. At the same time that the brain is receiving information from the nociceptors (the danger receptors that detect biological pain), the brain is also receiving visual, auditory, touch, movement, temperature and other information from the environment. The brain interprets the pain signals and gives meaning to them. Ultimately, the brain is trying to decide "is this dangerous or not?" However, the brain's interpretation is not always right — and it can also change.

There are various experiments with volunteers (yes, volunteers!) who go to a laboratory to feel pain as scientists study their brains and bodies. In one of these experiments, scientists applied the same painful stimulation at the same intensity, but they showed sad or happy pictures. Guess what? The volunteers felt more pain when they saw sad pictures and less pain when they saw happy pictures (Villemure and Bushnell, 2009).

But what about the people around us? Do we feel more intense pain if there is a loved one around or does that help to feel less intense pain? The answer is puzzling because it varies. It depends on the other person's empathy and perceived helpfulness. In the studies, it also depends how much trust and connection the volunteer patient feels toward the companion person.

HOLDING HANDS EASES THE PAIN

In a very interesting laboratory experiment, scientists invited couples in a romantic relationship to test a hypothesis (Goldstein et al., 2018). They wanted to test the ability of the brain to reduce the interpretation of pain by being comforted by a partner. The study involved 22 couples who were exposed to various painful stimulations. Their brain waves were also monitored using an electroencephalograph.

At first, the participants were sitting together in the same room without holding their hands. Then they were holding hands. Finally, they were put in separate rooms. Both males and females were exposed to painful stimulus while the other person was not. What they found was that their brain waves related to focus and attention were in synchrony when they were together. And this synchrony became even stronger if they held hands.

What was most interesting was that during the phase when the couples were holding hands, the person reported that their pain was a lot less intense.

Pain Is a Bio-Psycho-Social-Spiritual Matter

Our family, friends, community and society have much more influence over us than we think. Human beings are social and spiritual beings. People like to identify with their peers. They long for acceptance, forgiveness, gratitude, praise and belonging. Lonely and solitary people have the urge to connect with someone. Even if that person is a stranger they met on social media, someone that they would never meet in person, that person may have a strong influence on their beliefs, emotions and actions.

Who are the individuals in your support team? What are their roles? How do you reach to them when you need? How much have you disclosed to them about your chronic pain?

> Can you make a list of your support team? When you are having a bad pain day, who do you seek for support?

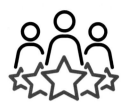

> Chronic pain is invisible. People cannot see your pain, and there is no way to prove that you are in pain. People with chronic pain tell me that they would prefer to have an amputation, cancer or a cardiac disease, so at least people would believe them and feel empathy for them.

How much do they know about the disease that you have? Yes, disease. The World Health Organization recognizes chronic pain as a disease and not just a symptom of something else (Treede et al., 2019).

Navigating chronic pain without a support team is a very lonely experience. What is most distressing is that many patients will prefer to hide their condition and diagnosis. They would rather speak with a stranger on a web-based discussion group than with their close relatives, coworkers or friends.

REASONS WHY PEOPLE PREFER NOT TO DISCLOSE THEIR CHRONIC PAIN

- "They would not know what to say or do."
- "They blame me for being in pain all the time."
- "They think I am a drug addict and all I want is pills."
- "They think I am faking pain to avoid work or chores."
- "They think I am weak and fragile."
- "They feel sorry for me, and it makes them sad."
- "They are tired of me complaining all the time."

Chronic pain is invisible. Many patients tell me they would rather have an amputation, a stroke or cancer, just so people would believe in their reports of pain.

> What is your main frustration with the people around you? Did you find a way to solve the problem of communicating about your pain with other people? I would love to hear about your solution. Use hashtag #ConquerPainWithDrFurlan on social media and let me know your thoughts.

How to Measure Pain

There is no thermometer to measure or prove pain. Pain is what a person says it is. Because chronic pain is different from acute pain, the measures should be different.

Acute pain from an injury or disease usually leads the person in pain to see a healthcare professional. The nurse or the doctor will assess the patient's situation and make a diagnosis. If the person has chest pain it could be esophageal reflux, a pulled muscle, angina or a myocardial infarct. If the person has knee pain it could be a fracture, ligament injury, gout attack or tendinitis.

They will usually ask the person to rate their pain on a scale from zero to 10, where zero is "no pain" and 10 is "the worst pain you can imagine." If the person answers 1 to 4 it is mild pain; 5 to 7 is moderate pain and 8 or above is high-intensity pain. Even for acute pain, this is not an accurate measure of how severe the injury or disease is. We saw in *What Is Pain?* that there are life-threatening situations, such as a stroke, where the person does not have any pain. And there are situations where the pain is unbearable in a body part that has been amputated.

With chronic pain, measuring pain is even more challenging. The numbers do not make much sense when someone is always, constantly in pain. For many, even when the pain is 4 out of 10, it is so tiring and annoying that it feels like 11 out of 10. Most of my patients would say that these questions do not make any sense to them, but unfortunately, we do not have a better method to assess pain intensity.

As mentioned in *Getting a Diagnosis*, I ask my patients to give me a number for the pain right now, the highest in the past seven days, the lowest in the past seven days and the average in the past seven days. Then I add all these scores and calculate a percentage out of 40, which would be the maximum.

The most common scenario among my patients with chronic pain is this:

Right now = 8
Highest = 10
Lowest = 5
Average = 8

Total score = 8 + 10 + 5 + 8 = 31/40 or 77.5%

WHY IS THIS PAIN RATING IMPORTANT?

- If we start any new treatment, or if we decide to stop any treatment the patient is receiving, we need to know if their perception of pain intensity is going up or down. Of course, we all want to see those numbers going down, but there are situations in which the pain will go up and we need to understand what is going on.
- If we can get more information about when the most pain and the least pain happen, we can understand better how to treat it. I use this information to ask patients "What makes your pain go from 10 to 5?"
- I want to understand how they cope when their pain is at the maximum, not at the lowest.
- I need to know if their pain is ever at a "zero." It gives me some hints if there is central sensitization and if the pain is nociplastic or not.

Talking about Pain with the People Who Are Close to Us

> "You don't know how much pain I have."
> "You don't understand me."
> "You are not helpful."

Communication with family members and those close to us is one of the major frustrations among people with chronic pain. Some of my patients have a relative who gets it, but many do not have that kind of person in their lives. I have heard over and over from patients that chronic pain destroyed their marriage, their relationships with their children and their friends.

These losses are deeply hurtful, and the person with chronic pain grieves and that makes their pain even worse. As we discussed in *Step 2: Control Your Emotions*, our emotions can make pain worse or better. The emotions that come from lost relationships can aggravate pain and amplify the suffering a hundred times.

People with chronic pain need to learn how to communicate with partners, family, friends and acquaintances.

It is important to keep family and friends around you to support you, but they also have their fears, needs and goals in life. They also need you to support them to become better people in this needy world. You are all in this together and destroying those relationships will not be helpful to you or to them.

SHELLEY, THE ACCOUNTANT WHO HAS NO PAIN WHEN SHE IS WORKING

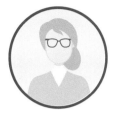 Shelley is a 70-year-old lady who has had two surgeries for a chronic back problem. She also has had both of her knees replaced, but still has pain in both knees, which has an impact on her ability to walk. She works full-time from home as an accountant. She loves her job, and she is not even thinking of retiring.

When I asked her the four questions to measure her pain, she gave me these numbers. Pain right now was 7.5; worst pain was 9.5; least pain was 0 and the average was 5.5.

I like to explore what makes the pain go up or down. It can be fascinating, as it was in Shelley's case!

She told me that when she was working, she concentrated on her clients and she didn't have any pain: her pain was zero. When she is not working, but just sitting on her sofa or in her car, her pain immediately returned to a 9.5.

What did that tell me? It told me that her brain was able to suppress the pain for many hours while she was distracted and not moving. She didn't feel pain at all then.

That was very good news. It meant we could work with her mind and body to bring about that state of zero pain more often.

We had to find out what was so different between work and home. She lived with her husband, who was very anxious and demanding. She has a daughter who is a lawyer and is always pressing the medical doctors to give more painkillers to her.

Shelley had difficulty saying no to her husband and her daughter, so she felt more in control at work than at home.

Shelley learned mindfulness and visualizations. Mindfulness helped her to feel the pain without fearing it. She had thought she would need more surgery to her back or her knees, but the visualizations helped her to relax her muscles, sleep better and reduce the worry about her knees and back.

She also lost weight, which reduced the chronic inflammation in her body and reduced the strain on her joints.

Below I have suggested nine tips to help you communicate better with family and friends. This is not an exhaustive list, and you may find more resources and solutions by talking to a social worker, a psychologist or other people with lived experiences of chronic pain who have conquered their chronic pain mountain.

NINE WAYS TO COMMUNICATE BETTER WITH FAMILY AND FRIENDS

1. Be clear about what you want
2. Avoid certain words
3. Ask for clarification
4. Be honest
5. Show respect
6. Accept their "no"
7. Be polite
8. Use humor
9. Do not play the victim

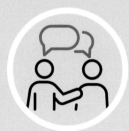

1. BE CLEAR ABOUT WHAT YOU WANT

If you need help with a task, or want someone to be by your side and listen, then just say that. Some people will send hidden messages and will expect their relative to get the message and do what they are expecting. We live in a world of text messages, emails and social media, where many people are losing the ability to communicate effectively.

Maybe you are sitting in the couch groaning and lamenting, trying to send the message that you want someone by your side reassuring you that you will be okay. But unless you communicate your wishes, the people around you won't necessarily know what you want. They may think that you want more painkillers or that you are depressed.

Your behavior may just push them away. They are probably willing to help, but if they offer something, they may be afraid that you are going to scream at them, saying, "You don't understand me!"

Consider the alternative. You could stop lamenting and say, "Honey, I just need you to hold my hands for a few minutes and reassure me that everything is all right, that I will improve, that I am a strong person. Can you do that for me? Can you help me to smile?"

2. AVOID CERTAIN WORDS

Avoid using words like "never" or "always," or saying "you don't understand me."

Sometimes we use strong words to convey strong emotions. Our words can heal or hurt. Once the words are out of our mouth, we cannot swallow them back. If we say something we regret, we can ask forgiveness and receive pardon, but spoken words are forever registered in the other person's brain.

Be very careful what you tell people, especially when you are in pain. Being in pain is not an excuse to say anything you want or anything that crosses your mind. Telling your romantic partner, "You never help me" is probably a lie. Or telling your children "You always make some excuse for not helping me" is also probably a lie. If you keep saying these things, your brain will believe them, and your relatives may also believe them and start behaving the way you say they are.

Have you been telling lies lately? What are some lies that you have told your family about them? Did you ever ask for forgiveness? It takes humility to do that, especially if you think that you are a victim.

3. ASK FOR CLARIFICATION

If your relative is not doing what you expect them to do, instead of blaming them and shaming them verbally, did you ask them about it?

Sometimes we make assumptions about people's reactions and reasoning, and those assumptions can be wrong.

If, for example, you asked your child to put the garbage out and they didn't, that means now you have to carry those heavy bags out in the middle of the winter and everyone knows that aggravates your back pain. You immediately assume they did this on purpose to hurt you, or that they forgot because they don't even care about you. When they get home, you shout at them and throws words like "You don't care about me."

Or you could try a better approach. When they arrive home, you can welcome them with a smile, start a normal conversation, ask how their day went, and then ask in a soft voice, "Did you forget to put the garbage out?"

4. BE HONEST

Be honest in your conversation. If your child answers "Yes, I forgot," you could show that you want to understand their side of the story. You may ask more questions, such as, "Are you worried about something at school that made you forget the garbage?"

You may tell them that you were a bit frustrated when you found that the garbage was still sitting at the side of the kitchen and that you brought it to the curbside. But that you are okay. You are not mad at them but you want to understand what can you do to help them remember next time.

Try putting yourself in their shoes. Their priorities are different from your priorities. Each person is concerned about their own affairs, and that is okay. There is nothing wrong with that, but living as a family involves some sharing of responsibilities and caring for each other. The only way to demonstrate this is by doing and modelling this.

5. SHOW RESPECT

If you show respect to the other person, to their responsibilities, concerns and goals in life, and you help them to achieve their own goals, they will naturally respond in a respectful way to you. If they do not, it might be because you have already built a high wall between you and them, and they can't find a way to penetrate the wall without breaking it.

Nurturing a romantic relationship is a daily task. You can't be rude and aggressive to your partner for years and then one day start changing your language and your behaviors and expect them to respond to your new attitude just as quickly. You may need marital counseling.

The same ideas apply to raising children. You need to respect them as a person even when they are just starting to babble and crawl. When I had my first child, a friend of mine gave me advice that I will never forget. She told me to treat my kids the same way that I would treat a very important guest at my house. Imagine this very important person is coming to dinner at your house tonight. What would you say? What words would you use? Would you be soft spoken or yelling at them? Would you receive them at the door with a smile or with whining and lamenting? Why would you treat your family members, your partner and your children differently than this so-called VIP?

Do you think that your spouse, children and parents do not notice when you treat them badly yet are sweet and polite with strangers? If you can be kind to strangers, why can't you do the same for them? Don't you think this is also frustrating them?

6. ACCEPT THEIR "NO"

What should we do when a family member we are asking for help says "no," or is not cooperating or not listening? What if they really don't care?

That happens more often than we think. It is sad to come across dysfunctional families. The disease of chronic pain may be one of the factors that contributes to family problems, but there are many other reasons for this to happen. For the person living with chronic pain, hearing a "no" can feel like a punch in the face. The problem is that this emotion will trigger the brain centers of anger, frustration, fear and sadness. All these are emotions that are highly connected to the pain areas in the brain and will probably lead to a flare-up.

So, what is the solution to hearing a "no"? There are many possibilities, and you have to figure out which responses work best for you. The first thing you need to do is hear the "no" clearly. Was it a firm no or a temporary no? Some people will say things that offend you in the moment, but later they will regret them and be sorry. That may be a temporary "no." If what you heard was a firm "no," consider your reaction to that and what you are going to do about it.

"If you show respect to the other person, to their responsibilities, concerns and goals in life, and you help them to achieve their own goals, they will naturally respond in a respectful way to you."

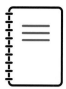

Advise yourself

Let's do an exercise.

1 Get two pieces of paper. Label them *1. My thoughts and feelings* and *2. My counsel to myself.*

2 On the first page, write down your thoughts and feelings toward a family member who is making your life miserable. Write down what you would like to tell that person. You are not writing a letter to them. They will not see what you are writing. This is just to help you to understand your own thoughts and emotions at that moment.

3 Now, on the second page, write a letter to yourself. Imagine you are a counselor who is giving advice to you at this moment. What would that counselor say to you?

4 Throw the first page out and keep the second with you. Use it when you need a reminder.

7. BE POLITE

Do not use harsh words toward others or to yourself. You can feel the difference when you change your language. Here are some examples:

AVOID THIS	INSTEAD, USE THIS
I hate when you look at me with pity.	It makes me sad when you look at me with pity.
You obviously do not know how to help me.	I noticed that when I need help, you try your best, but I understand it is hard to know how to help me in this situation.
She is selfish; she cares only about herself.	She has her own problems and frustrations, and she needs time and space to figure out how she will solve them.
He thinks I am a drug addict.	He loves me. He is concerned about me and how I am using these painkillers.
He blames me because I smoke and am fat and lazy.	He is trying to help me change my bad habits. He wants to motivate me, but he doesn't know how to do this properly.

Change your language

Let's do another writing exercise.

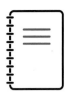

Think about some phrases that you have been using to describe your family members or friends in the past week, month or years. You may feel bad to be thinking negative things about your own family and friends, but you need to be honest with yourself.

1. Get two pieces of paper.

2. On the first page, write down exactly what you say to your family or friends on a regular basis. Or write what you tell other people about them, or what you think about them even if you don't tell others. Include their names. Again, they will not see what you are writing. This is just to help you to understand your thoughts and emotions.

3. Now, on the second page, rewrite those sentences using more balanced, polite language.

4. Throw the first page out and keep the second with you. Read the messages on that second page every day until your brain believes these messages.

8. USE HUMOR

Living with chronic pain is not a reason to lose your sense of humor. Being in good humor is a state of mind and a choice. When you are in good humor, you may feel cheerful, agreeable and generally in a positive mood.

Bad humor may look like irritability, grumpiness or depression. But bad humor is not the same as being depressed. Depression is a serious medical condition that is characterized by feelings of sadness, emptiness and hopelessness.

Science has shown that having a good sense of humor is beneficial to our health. As humans, we use humor, especially spoken language, to amuse others and ourselves. There are short-term benefits to laughter: it relieves stress and muscle tension and stimulates production of endorphins, our own feel-good medicine. In the long term, a person who has a good sense of humor has less pain, better moods, a better immune system and better personal relationships with other people.

As it says in the Bible, "A cheerful heart is good medicine, but a crushed spirit dries up the bones" (Proverbs 17:22).

Is it possible to develop a good sense of humor, or is humor a genetic or personality trait?

Both statements are true. It is possible to learn, but it can also be a personality trait and depend on cultural norms. There are self-help books, videos, coaching courses and mentors that provide training to people who want to improve in this area and practice their skills.

It is important to keep in mind that forcing humor is not super helpful. It has to be genuine and spontaneous. Also, trying to be too "funny" may not be the correct response in some situations when there is really sadness and loss, as with a diagnosis of a terminal disease. We should be careful not to offend others' feelings by making jokes about their ethnicity, color, education, physical deformities or religion. It is important to understand the cultural context in which humor can be expressed and how much of it is acceptable in that context.

9. DO NOT PLAY THE VICTIM

A person with chronic pain may see themselves as a victim. They may seek attention in the form of pity from the people around them. This is common in those who have chronic pain because of a trauma such as a car crash, a work-related injury or a personal assault. There are a couple of problems with this situation.

First, you may get the attention and things that you want because those around you feel sorry for your suffering and want to compensate you for that. While it is nice to get all we want from the people we love, you just need to complain a little and everything is given to you. In other words, you don't need to make too much effort to get what you want. You can become spoiled by this. Because of this, your life may feel empty of worth and you can end up being trapped, having to play the role of a sick person to get what you want. And people around you will get tired and upset because you are getting away with minimal effort while they are making sacrifices to help you.

The second problem is that playing the victim really gets into your head and you end up believing that you are a victim. Therefore, any attempt to reverse that situation will be faced with resistance.

I commonly see this behavior in people who retain legal counsel to help them win a process against a person or a company that is responsible for their chronic pain or their suffering. For them to win the legal case, they need to demonstrate they are a victim of some injustice or neglect.

This behavior is also common among people who receive financial compensation for their chronic pain, as in a workers compensation case. The person may unconsciously believe they need to play the victim to continue receiving their payments.

The problem with this behavior is that any attempt to retrain the pain system and eliminate pain is faced with resistance. The brain is in conflict.

CASE STUDY

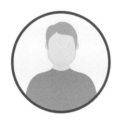

PRINCE, THE SPOILED BOY

Prince was 28 years old the first time I met him. He had had several health issues since childhood, and his family did everything they could to provide him with a good life. From the time he was 12 years old, he had complained of pain all over his body. His family tried all kinds of expensive treatments for him, but nothing worked.

There is nothing wrong with a family demonstrating love and supporting a member of the family who is in need. However, some families and friends are enablers of disability. In this case, this young man got all he needed from his family without making any effort for himself.

We needed to find something that would motivate Prince to step out of his role as a helpless sick person. We spent a lot of time coaching him. We worked with his family to help them see him as a grown-up man and to give him responsibility for his own care and well-being.

Since then, he has taken on a part-time job and is opening his own business. He is no longer a victim.

Communicating Pain to Your Doctor

At some point in your journey, maybe often, you will have to explain your chronic pain to a doctor, your physiotherapist or another member of your healthcare team.

There are various types of doctors you can talk to about your pain.

Primary care

In many places in the world, the patient has a primary care clinician. This person can be a family doctor, a nurse practitioner, a physiotherapist or a physician assistant.

Primary care means these clinicians offer a spectrum of services beyond the traditional healthcare system. They assist with health promotion, injury prevention, diagnosis and treatment of illnesses. Physicians who work in primary care facilities have a long-term relationship with their patients, usually for years, so they know their patients very well. But they do not have much time to spend with patients at every visit.

Emergency departments

Many patients with chronic pain do not have access to primary care or pain specialists, and they end up in emergency departments, as in a hospital or a community clinic.

The professionals working in emergency services do not have much time to spend with patients. They are more concerned with helping the patient who has a life-threatening problem at the moment.

Pain doctors

Pain doctors are experts in helping people who have chronic pain. Pain doctors may work by themselves or at a pain clinic as part of a multidisciplinary team, as I do. We discussed pain doctors in an earlier chapter, *Getting a Diagnosis*.

Stigma about Taking Opioids for Chronic Pain

We discussed the questions a doctor or pain clinician will ask you in an initial interview in *Getting a Diagnosis.* By the time you get to a pain specialist, you may have already tried various kinds of painkillers. Your next hurdle could be talking to this new doctor about opioids — maintaining, eliminating or starting them.

People who use opioids for pain often complain they feel stigma at many levels. Their family and friends view them as weak and vulnerable. Their doctors suspect they are abusing and addicted to opioids, and the pharmacists who dispense their medications them treat them as if they are selling these pills to make extra cash.

Many patients are afraid of talking about opioids with their doctors. They are afraid of being judged, criticized and stereotyped. Opioids are the most powerful painkillers and there are still many people who use them for pain management.

A few decades ago, doctors were persuaded to prescribe opioids to anyone with pain. Now, they are being pushed to stop prescribing opioids for pain. No wonder there is a lot of confusion and mistrust.

Patients who are caught in the middle of this opioid crisis have a serious problem. If they are receiving opioids to manage their pain, how should they respond if the doctor suggests stopping their opioids? How will that conversation go? Or, if they have not been prescribed opioids and they are in severe pain, what should they tell their doctors to initiate a trial of opioid therapy to test if they are responsive to this type of medication?

> Stigma is when someone judges you in a negative way based on some characteristics that you present. It could be the color of your skin, your accent, some visible physical difference or a mental health condition.

Talking to your doctor about opioid tapering

If you have been receiving opioids for chronic pain, your body is pretty much accustomed to them. That is what we call **physical dependence**. Your body does not like it when you miss a dose of opioids. That is what we call **withdrawal symptoms**. All that you know is that, even if you still have pain, you need these opioids to keep a sense of a normal life.

You are worried because your doctor has suggested that they will not continue to prescribe your opioids anymore.

WATCH MY VIDEO ON HOW TO TALK TO YOUR DOCTOR ABOUT OPIOIDS

This might be because your doctor has decided they will not keep prescribing opioids to you anymore or because they are retiring or moving practice. What can you say at your next appointment?

This appointment will not be easy. I advise you to prepare for this difficult conversation. I have been in this situation myself, many times, when I have had to inform a patient that I was not going to prescribe their opioids anymore. And I had reasons for tapering and stopping that prescription. Here are some thoughts to help you prepare for that conversation:

1. Remember that you are responsible for what you say and what you do. Do not say or do anything that you will regret later, such as being rude or impolite.

2. Explain the reasons why you have been taking opioids. Talk about your symptoms before you were put on opioids and what changed in your life after you started taking them.

3. Talk about any previous attempts to reduce the dose or to stop taking the opioids. What happened and how was it done? Did you try to stop cold turkey? Did you try a slow taper? Did you try medications to manage the withdrawal symptoms?

4. If the dose has to be reduced, ask about a plan to manage the withdrawal symptoms. How will you get help if there are intense symptoms? Where should you go and who could help you? Is there a nurse, a pharmacist or clinic staff you can call? How long will it take? You may ask for a slow taper.

5. If possible, try to get a second opinion with a pain specialist before stopping opioids. There are some interventions and other treatments that can help your pain and the need for opioids. Some opioids, such as buprenorphine and methadone, have fewer withdrawal symptoms, and maybe the pain doctor could help you get those.

> What do you find most difficult when talking to your physician about pain? I would love to hear. Tag me with #ConquerPainWithDrFurlan on social media.

Talking to your doctor about starting opioids

The second scenario is if you have never received opioids and you have severe pain that is very debilitating for you. Perhaps you wonder why your doctor has never suggested opioid therapy. You would like to hear about the benefits and risks of this therapy. How do you open up that discussion without sounding like a drug seeker who is looking to get high on these powerful opioids?

I suggest you prepare a list of your questions for when you talk with your doctor. Following are some examples.

1. At your next appointment, ask the doctor if your pain is responsive to opioids. There are some pain conditions that do not respond well to opioids. For example, with nociplastic pain, your pain may get worse with opioids. See pages 200–202 in *Step 6: Check Your Medicine Cabinet*.

2. Ask the doctor if you can try a low dose of opioid therapy as a trial. At the end of the trial period, usually three months, you and the doctor will decide if the trial was successful or not.

3. Ask your doctor if they are concerned about any risks you may have in relation to opioids. Are they concerned about addiction, overdose or other complications? These other complications might be sleep apnea, immunosuppression, low sex hormones, osteoporosis, risks of falls or risk of sleepiness that could cause a car accident or at work.

4. Ask about the maximum dose that you will be taking on a daily basis. It is important that you and the doctor agree on a maximum dosage, an approximate number that the doctor will not prescribe above, so you will not be surprised later. For example, you may choose not to go above 100 mg of morphine equivalents per day.

5. If you are a female patient and of reproductive age, ask your doctor if there is a plan for stopping the opioid when you get pregnant, because opioids cross the placenta and there is a risk of neonatal abstinence syndrome, which can seriously affect the health of the baby.

6. Ask your doctor what happens if they are not available to renew your prescriptions. What if they go on vacation, or get sick? Who will replace them and is that other doctor going to renew your prescriptions on time?

The Role of the Community Pharmacist in Your Pain Management

> Pharmacists are trained to provide care to patients and counseling regarding their use of medications.

Pharmacists are health professionals with expertise in the preparation, uses of and interactions between medications. They are trained to provide care to patients and counseling regarding their use of medications. They are regulated by a professional college and they can refuse to dispense any medication that they consider unsafe to the patient. They may contact the prescribing physician and ask for adjustments or modifications of doses and types of medications.

Pharmacists have access to computerized databases that physicians usually do not have, and these databases may inform of relevant interactions between diverse medications. For example, a patient may not tell their doctor that they are receiving medication from another doctor. The pharmacist has all information about the client in one place, and they can check for interactions that may occur among different medications.

In some jurisdictions where there is a narcotic monitoring program, pharmacists have access to information about all narcotics that the patient has received, even if at other pharmacies. Then, the pharmacists may suggest adjustments in the quantities that the patient will receive. In some situations, when patients are prescribed high doses of opioids, the pharmacy may decide to dispense a smaller amount at a shorter interval.

There are situations when a patient may lose control of their use of opioids. For example, they will use many opioids in the first few days after they get their supply, and then not have enough to last the entire month. To avoid this problem, the doctor and pharmacist may decide that the patient can only get their supply for one week at a time or, in severe cases, they need to go to the pharmacy every day. In very serious cases, they will need to swallow the medication every day in the presence of the pharmacist.

Pharmacists can also counsel patients about over-the-counter medications that do not need a doctor's prescriptions. They are also very knowledgeable about topical creams and applications such as heat and cold as well as solutions to counter the side effects of chronic pain medications. (See *Step 6: Check Your Medicine Cabinet.*)

CHUCK WAS PICKING UP 1,440 OXYCODONE TABLETS AT THE PHARMACY

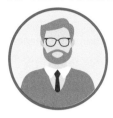

Chuck is a 42-year-old male with chronic pain after a spinal cord injury that left him paraplegic. He was prescribed eight tablets per day of an opioid, oxycodone immediate release. His family doctor sees him every six months and renews his prescription then.

He was getting 1,440 tablets of oxycodone, all at one time, every six months at the pharmacy. To give you an idea of what that looks like, imagine a plastic grocery bag full of tablets. That is too much to take home and to store at home. As these pills, like heroin or cocaine, have a street value, he could be assaulted and robbed when leaving the pharmacy.

For Chuck's health and safety, we suggested his pharmacist dispense 240 tablets once a month. And, as usual, we recommended he keep his opioids in a locked cabinet at home, and away from children, teenagers and guests.

Chuck hadn't realized that this system of dispensing his medication was problematic, but he was happy with our solution, as was his pharmacist.

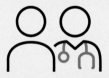

"Collaborations between doctors and pharmacists should be the norm, not the exception."

Peer-Support Groups

It is important to recognize healthy support groups as opposed to toxic groups. A healthy conversation can point you in the right direction to get better, to overcome your barriers and they share success stories. In toxic groups, the tone of the discussion is usually demeaning, depressing and violent.

A support group that is composed by people with lived experiences of the same condition as you have can be very helpful and enlightening. These groups are usually organized by people who were able to overcome their conditions and now they volunteer to organize regular sessions with people newly diagnosed with that health condition. Some of these groups meet in person, while others using videoconferences or discuss topics using social media platforms.

I recommend my patients connect with organizations that are well established and have a governing body such as a chair, a moderator and an advisory board that oversees their activities. There are various not-for-profit organizations and foundations that offer a platform for patients to have discussions and help each other.

Check the *References and Resources* section of this book for some associations in Canada, the United States and other countries that offer services for people with chronic pain.

Managers, Coworkers and Human Resources

Some chronic pain conditions may affect your ability to work, and some medications prescribed for pain may impair your coordination and concentration. These factors may affect how effectively and safely you can perform some activities at work.

You need to consider disclosing your health condition at work and requesting modified duties or modified hours. There are benefits and risks to disclosing your pain diagnosis at work.

Many patients hide their pain at work and then suffer the consequences at home, by being exhausted and using their vacation days as sick days. Individuals who are self-employed or work on contract or in a small business usually do not have the benefits of a workplace that offers accommodations or modified duties. They can either work or not work. Individuals who work for a large employer, one that offers work modifications and accommodations, usually find it easier to disclose a health condition.

Many patients do not want to disclose their chronic pain because they are waiting for their pain to resolve or disappear. The longer they wait while the pain does not resolve, the more frustrated, depressed and fearful they become. They worry that they will lose their job and will be unable to provide for their families. The advantage of disclosing early is that you may be able to work with less pain and therefore be more productive.

Disclosing your chronic pain to a trusted co-worker can be helpful if you explain the nature of your pain and co-create a contingency plan with them. They will know what to expect from day to day. They may be prepared to fill in for you on days when you can't work.

MODIFICATIONS AND ACCOMMODATIONS

The following are the most common employment modifications requested for people with chronic pain.

- *Modified hours:* Some patients need to attend sessions of physiotherapy, counselling or other kinds of therapies. If these sessions are offered only during work hours, the patient may need flexible hours to start and finish their work so they can attend these therapy sessions.
- *Modified activities:* These may include changes in the physical requirements, such as sitting on a stool instead of standing for longer hours.
- *Accommodations for using certain drug treatments:* Some patients are prescribed medications such as opioids, muscle relaxants or cannabinoids that can impair their concentration or coordination. If their work involves use of heavy equipment or driving a motor vehicle, they need accommodations to avoid any injury or trauma to themselves or to other people.
- *Working from home:* Thanks to modern technology, connecting to work remotely gives many patients the flexibility to set up their own workplace and avoid long commutes.

Insurance and Workers' Compensation

Sometimes chronic pain begins as a result of acute trauma in a motor vehicle collision or a work-related injury. When this is the case, an adjudicator will decide if the patient is entitled to compensation. This compensation may include reimbursement for all treatment related to that condition and, in some cases, salary compensation for lost income.

Patients need to open a claim with their insurance, either their car insurance or their workers' compensation board. The documentation and forms can be overwhelming at first, and many patients retain legal counsel or paralegal services to assist with all paperwork.

It is important that you keep good notes of your medical appointments and complete all forms required by your insurance. Your doctor and other members of your healthcare team may be asked to provide medical information about you. You need to authorize your healthcare professional to release your medical information to your insurance or workers' compensation.

Legal Counsel

Legal and paralegal services are helpful if the person has chronic pain because of an accident-related injury and they require assistance to obtain compensation or access to medical care. If you are in any doubt, it is always better to consult legal counsel.

The type of compensation the person is eligible for varies depending on the type of insurance and also in different provinces, states and countries. The types of compensation generally fall under these categories:

- Compensation for the lost income due to their inability to perform their duties at work
- Access to medical and rehabilitation care
- Remuneration related to pain and suffering

I am so proud of you! You made it to this point.
You have learned so much. Are you practicing what you learned?
Are you enjoying the activities so far?
Tag me on social media using the hashtag
#ConquerPainWithDrFurlan.

CONCLUSION

By now, you have probably realized that the people around you have a lot of influence on the pain that you feel. The way you interact and communicate with other people may ease your pain or make it worse.

In this chapter, I have provided you with some tips on how to communicate with partners, family members, friends, healthcare professionals, coworkers and managers, and what to expect from these interactions. You may need to come back to this chapter from time to time and refresh your memory on some points.

KEY POINTS TO REMEMBER

- Conquering pain is a team effort; you need to get help from other people.
- Empathy is a phenomenon that occurs in the brain. People are wired to feel each other's pain.
- Pain is not just a biological matter; it is a bio-psycho-social-spiritual matter. The social component is very important.
- Learn how to communicate effectively about pain with family, friends and acquaintances.
- Learn how to communicate about your pain and your medications, especially about opioids, which can be a very stigmatizing and challenging conversation.
- The doctors, nurses, community pharmacist, pain specialists and clinics and peer-support groups can all have a role in helping you manage your pain.
- Work is important, and so is your productivity. Disclosing your pain to managers, coworkers and human resources may help you to continue working and get you some financial assistance.

LOOKING AHEAD

In the next chapter, *Step 6: Check Your Medicine Cabinet,* we look inside your medicine cabinet and examine the options available to you. We talk about anti-inflammatories, opioids, antidepressants, antiepileptics and cannabinoids. We discuss how much pain relief to expect with medications for chronic pain.

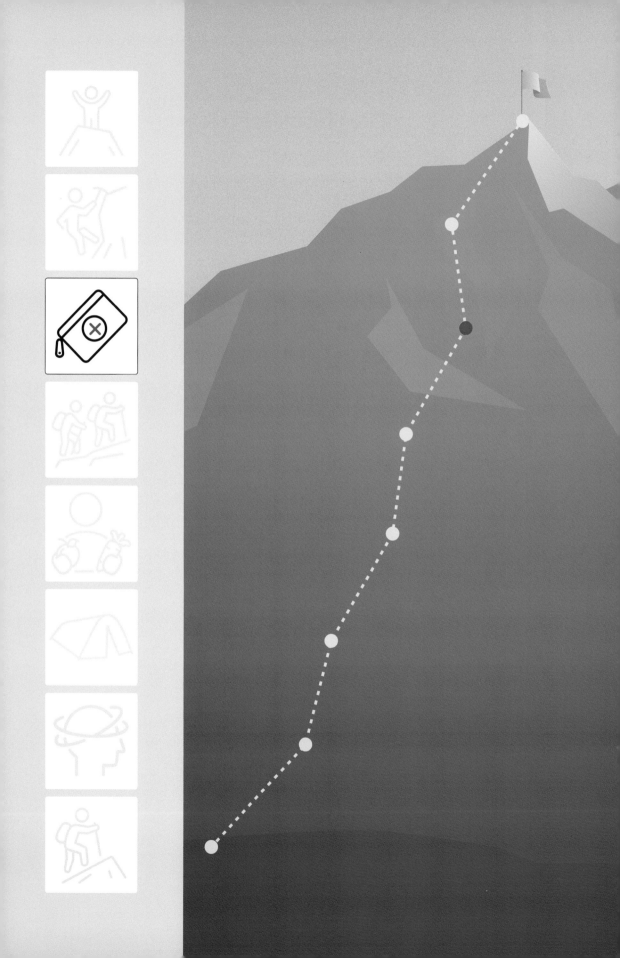

STEP 6

Check Your Medicine Cabinet

Imagine on the third week of the journey up the mountain, a severe storm hits. The climber's clothing and gear become wet and heavy; it is difficult to see the way ahead and the rocks are slippery. It is hard to keep focused. It is hard to think of anything else. The mountaineer needs a break.

When pain becomes unbearable, life gets hard and you see no way out but to resort to the medicine cabinet, open a bottle and take the pill. After all, they are called painkillers, right? They offer a quick solution to your suffering. But should you?

The journey to conquer pain is not a straight line going up. There will be good days and bad days. If possible, my preference is to manage chronic pain without pain medications, or with the least amount necessary or for the shortest possible period. But it is okay to use medications if you need them, especially to get you through a bad day.

In this chapter, we discuss how important it is to keep track of your medications and regularly review their effectiveness. I'll introduce you to your pain medications team. And I'll explain how the types of medications we use to treat chronic pain are different from the ones we use to treat acute pain.

You'll also see how not all painkillers kill pain. We consider reasons why you may want to avoid using pain medications. We talk about the different kinds of prescription medications used to treat chronic pain and what to expect from them. And finally, we consider other options, including medications that do not need a doctor's prescription.

What's in Your Medicine Cabinet?

Your doctor may have already prescribed opioids, antidepressants, antiepileptics and/or cannabinoids for your chronic pain. Each of these options has their benefits and drawbacks. (For more about these prescription medications, see pages 204–209.)

There are also medications that don't need a doctor's prescription, including over-the-counter (OTC) medications such as ibuprofen, acetaminophen, some muscle relaxants and topical creams. These drugs are sold in pharmacies, grocery shops and department stores. They are not as safe as they seem. (For more about OTC medications, see page 209.)

It's possible you take certain diet supplements, such as magnesium, to relieve your chronic pain. (For more about these, see pages 131 and 152.)

If you do not use any pain medication and do not have any pills at home, you will still want to continue reading this chapter. There are some drugs that your doctor may offer to you in the form of an injection or intravenous infusion. Also, your doctor may want you to consider a trial of some medication to relieve your pain.

Polypharmacy

Some patients take multiple medications for pain, both prescribed and over-the counter. We call this polypharmacy. There are some cases where polypharmacy makes sense, but there many other instances when the combinations and sheer number of medications a person takes is irrational and even dangerous.

MR. BOTTLES AND HIS MANY PAIN PILLS

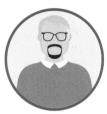 A family doctor sent me a referral asking my opinion about a patient with chronic low back pain, arthritis, headaches and neuropathic pain. I am calling him "Mr. Bottles" for a good reason.

He was 93 years old and came with his wife of more than 60 years. Before retiring, he used to be a tennis player and coach, so he had always been very physically active and fit. Now, he was not doing any physical activity except walking, and his only strategy to manage his pain was taking medications.

He was taking two different non-steroidal anti-inflammatory drugs (NSAIDs), ibuprofen and celecoxib, three different opioids (codeine, hydromorphone and transdermal fentanyl), two antidepressants (amitriptyline and duloxetine), two antiepileptic drugs (gabapentin and topiramate) and one sedative (lorazepam).

He brought a plastic bag containing bottles of all the medications he takes daily. I could not fit all the bottles on the top of my desk. And his wife told me there were more bottles at home that he didn't bring.

What this case illustrates is a desperation to get rid of pain. He and his family doctor were believers that more medication was the solution. But it was not. He was taking all of that and was still in pain.

We started a de-prescribing plan for him. Our clinic's pharmacist got involved and, as we began reducing the daily pills and patches, "Mr. Bottles" started a routine of daily exercises. His pain improved dramatically, and we discharged him with only three tablets per day for his pain.

"More is not always better."

Review all of your pain medications

Let's do an exercise.

① Get out your journal and make a list of all your pain medications, filling in the information noted below. See the case study on the facing page for an example.

DRUG OR BRAND NAME	WHAT CLASS OF MEDICATION IS IT?	WHICH PAIN DOES IT TREAT?	HOW IS IT WORKING?	DOES IT CAUSE ANY ADVERSE EFFECTS?

Drug name is the name of the molecule; this could be codeine, morphine, duloxetine, pregabalin, gabapentin, acetaminophen, etc.

Brand name is the trade name given by the pharmaceutical company that patented the drug; this could be Tylenol, Cymbalta, Lyrica, Neurontin, etc.

Class of medication refers to the action of the drug. Is it an analgesic, anti-inflammatory, anticonvulsant, antidepressant, cannabinoid, local anesthetic, etc.

How is it working? You may record if it is helping or not with the pain, what happens when you take it, how much improvement do you notice on your pain.

Adverse effects: Here the list can be very long, but do you notice anything unpleasant or any undesirable effect of the drug on your body?

② Look at your list and answer these questions:

- Do you know what each medication does to your pain and to your health?
- How much pain relief are you supposed to expect from each drug?
- Are you sure they are not causing more harm than benefit?

It is important that you know what you are taking and the purpose of each medication, so you and you pain care team can know if they are working. That is why I ask my patients to complete a list of their medications like this one.

LARRY KNOWS WHY HE TAKES WHAT HE TAKES FOR PAIN

 Larry was a 59-year-old landscape gardener. I asked him to complete a list of his medications. Here is what he gave me:

DRUG OR BRAND NAME	WHAT CLASS OF MEDICATION IS IT?	WHICH PAIN DOES IT TREAT?	HOW IS IT WORKING?	DOES IT CAUSE ANY ADVERSE EFFECTS?
Pregabalin	Antiepileptic	Pain in the legs from spinal stenosis	I still have pain in the legs when I walk. I didn't notice much difference since I started on pregabalin.	Trouble concentrating. Gained 10 pounds
Tramadol	Opioid and antidepressant	Lower back pain	When pain is unbearable, I take one tablet and pain improves 50%. I only use two to three times a week.	Dry mouth

After seeing this information, and some discussion, I suggested that Larry stop pregabalin and keep tramadol. (For more about what these medications do, see pages 204 and 206.)

Larry lost the weight he had gained on pregabalin and he also feels more alert during the day, which was important because he works with sharp tools and heavy equipment. His pain didn't get much worse. He continues using tramadol up to three times a week and that helps him on a hard day.

He downloaded a relaxation app to his smartphone, so when his pain is bad, he goes to his truck and practices relaxation for 15 minutes. He says that helps to calm down his anxiety about this pain and, in turn, his pain is less troublesome to him.

The combination of a change to his medications and practicing relaxation exercises has helped to relieve his pain.

Do Painkillers Really Kill the Pain?

In medical school, we learn a lot about medications, and that is why medical doctors like to use them. You may remember from the chapter *What Is Pain?* that there are three kinds of pain. (If you need a refresher, turn to pages 28–30.) Depending on the type of pain, painkillers can help or they can worsen the pain.

Nociceptive pain is when the pain system is doing what it is supposed to do, alerting your brain that there is an injury or disease in the periphery that needs to be fixed, like a bone fracture or appendicitis. Painkillers are excellent for eliminating this kind of pain. You can use anti-inflammatories, muscle relaxants, acetaminophen or opioids.

For *neuropathic pain,* in the early hours or days after a nerve injury, medications such as antidepressants and anticonvulsants may work very well to reduce the electrical activity of the nerves and reduce the pain. Although they are not usually called "painkillers," they reduce pain by reducing neuronal activity, both in the nerves and in the brain.

When there is *nociplastic pain,* opioids do not work the way they are designed to. Because the pain system is malfunctioning, the opioids do not have the expected effects, as in the case when there is no neuroplasticity of the pain system. Initially, when a person starts taking opioids, they feel pain relief, which is the result of the medications working in the areas of the pain system that are still intact. However, when opioids get to the areas of the pain system that are malfunctioning, as in central sensitization, the effects are quite the opposite; they amplify the pain signals arriving at the brain. This phenomenon is called *opioid-induced hyperalgesia* (see page 201).

FAQ

If these pills I've heard about are called painkillers, it must be for a good reason. Do they really kill the pain?

• •

Not all types of chronic pain respond well to painkillers. Depending on the type of pain, some medications commonly prescribed for pain can either help or make the pain worse.

If you are being discharged from hospital with a prescription for pain medications, the pharmacist at the hospital can communicate with the pharmacist in the community to provide information about changes that happened while you were in hospital.

The Pain Medication Team

Your healthcare team includes many clinicians. The medication triad team includes the doctor, the pharmacist and the nurse. These three professionals should be included in decisions regarding starting, maintaining and stopping medications. We have already discussed the roles of the interprofessional pain team in *Step 5: Get Help from Others.*

The doctor will diagnose which kind of pain you have. Is it nociceptive, neuropathic or nociplastic? They will check the evidence from randomized trials, meta-analyses and clinical practice guidelines. The doctor knows your other health issues and will suggest the best medication for you. At this point, the pharmacist should be consulted to provide information about interactions with other drugs you take for other conditions. The nurse is readily available to answer questions about when and how to take these medications; they can be your coach and also provide you with strategies to minimize side effects.

Measuring Pain and Function Before and After a Trial of Pain Medication

Your doctor may ask you to do a trial of a medication they think will help you and then reassess your pain and function after a couple of months to see if there is any improvement. (For more about measuring pain, see page 44 and page 163.)

When you do a trial of a medication, we need to find out if the medication is working or not, so we can decide if we will continue or not.

How do we know if there have been benefits or not? Asking a person to remember if their pain got better or not is tricky, because human beings have a hard time remembering how much pain they had in the past. They remember how they felt, but remembering the intensity is difficult.

TECHNICAL TERMS

A *randomized trial* is an experiment in which scientists randomly assign some people to receive one type of treatment and another group to receive a different type of treatment.

A *meta-analysis* combines multiple studies into one single statistical analysis.

This is because we have a protective mechanism in our memory to allow us to forget how bad pain was. Take, for example, a child who is learning how to walk. They will fall hundreds of times before they master this skill. Each time they fall, they feel pain, but they must forget how it feels. Otherwise, babies would become crawling adults who are afraid of walking.

To get a more accurate perspective of how much benefit a pain medication, or any other pain treatment, is providing, we collect some information before and after a trial period. We've already discussed the questionnaires I give patients when I first meet them, including the one in which they rate their pain.

Measuring pain

Remember? Zero is no pain, and 10 is the most excruciating pain that you can imagine.

We compare the total rating before with the total after trialing the medication. Is there a reduction in the total score? The maximum is 40. A 4-point drop is 10 percent. We consider any drop of 30 percent or higher a significant drop.

SEVERITY

0	2	4	6	8	10

Right now _____

Highest 7 days _____

Lowest 7 days _____

Average 7 days _____

Let's say it was 36/40 before and now it is 20/40. There was a drop of 16 points. In terms of percentage, this is 16 points out of 40, which is 16/40 times 100. That equals a drop of 40 percent.

That is a significant drop.

Measuring function

Pain is not the only factor that we want to improve with pain medication. It is also important to increase your functional levels. You can measure your function using a few simple questions.

On a scale from 0 (does not interfere) to 10 (completely interferes), you can rate how much pain interferes with these activities: general activity, mood, walking ability, normal work, relations with other people, sleep and enjoyment of life. In this rating, a lower number is better.

The maximum is 70 points. A drop of 21 points is equivalent to 30 percent. That would be a significant improvement.

FUNCTION

Rate how much pain interferes with these functions.

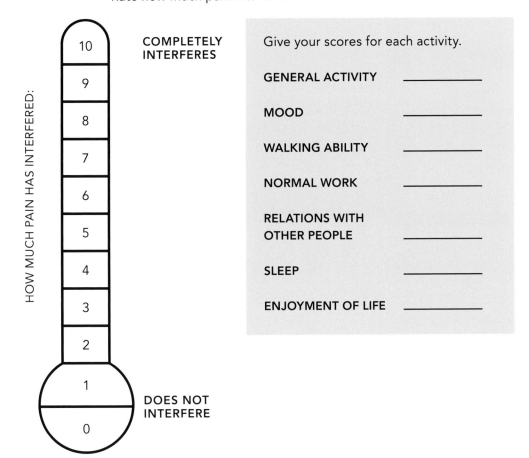

HOW MUCH PAIN HAS INTERFERED:

10 — COMPLETELY INTERFERES
9
8
7
6
5
4
3
2
1 — DOES NOT INTERFERE
0

Give your scores for each activity.

GENERAL ACTIVITY _____

MOOD _____

WALKING ABILITY _____

NORMAL WORK _____

RELATIONS WITH OTHER PEOPLE _____

SLEEP _____

ENJOYMENT OF LIFE _____

How Much Relief from Chronic Pain Can You Expect from Medications?

The amount of pain relief you get from medications can depend on the origin of your pain. The same drug has different effects when used to treat an acute pain of a nociceptive origin or a chronic pain of nociplastic or neuropathic origin.

For example, opioids are very potent and may completely eliminate pain when given to ease acute pain caused by a surgical incision. However, if the person develops chronic post-surgical pain, which is a type of mixed neuropathic and nociplastic chronic pain, then the opioid that was used to treat the acute post-surgical pain will not have the same effects for the chronic pain. In the case of acute pain, we can expect close to 100 percent pain relief. But with chronic pain, we are happy when we achieve around 30 percent pain relief.

It is difficult for someone who is already using opioids to know exactly what their pain is without opioids. If they take daily opioids for months, or years, how are they expected to know how much pain relief they have? They can't abruptly stop their painkillers to see what happens to their pain, because that will cause withdrawal symptoms, and one of the main symptoms of opioid withdrawal is pain all over the body.

Duration of Treatment

> Tapering means reducing the dose of the medication slowly to avoid withdrawal symptoms.

One question that patients frequently ask me is how long they will need to take their pain medications. This is hard to answer. Chronic pain is a chronic disease.

It is quite logical for patients to conclude that if the drugs help their pain, they will need to take them for the rest of their lives. Other people decide to stop because they are not happy with the side effects or the lack of benefits. They expected more from their pills and they are disappointed with the results, so they quit.

There are situations where the patient needs only one type of pain medication, and they use a low dose for many months or years. We may need to revisit their situation in a couple of years and opt to taper (gradually reduce the dosage) and stop to see what happens.

Is it safe to take these medications for many years?

All drugs have side effects and all of them lead to some changes in body functions. It would be much better not to take any medication, but that is unrealistic for some patients.

I don't recommend that patients read the list of all potential side effects that can occur with the drugs they are taking. That can trigger anxiety and a psychological reaction causing your brain to make you think you are having all the side effects that you read about in the drug monograph. This is what we call the "nocebo" effect.

Nevertheless, it is important that you mention your concerns to your pain team, especially the clinicians in the medication triad: the physician, pharmacist or nurse. The nurse is usually more readily available to answer questions you have about any adverse side effects, and they are very knowledgeable about what strategies you can use to manage and minimize side effects and continue taking the medications. The table below shows some examples:

MEDICATION FOR PAIN	SIDE EFFECT	MANAGING THE SIDE EFFECT
Opioids	Constipation	Stool softeners or laxatives
	Nausea	Ginger or antiemetics
	Itchiness	Antiallergy medications
Antidepressants	Insomnia	Magnesium, melatonin, sleep hygiene or sleeping aids
	Dry mouth	Lip gels and balms
Non-steroidal anti-inflammatory drugs (NSAIDs)	Stomach upset	Anti-acid medications

WHY ARE DOCTORS ALWAYS PUSHING ME TO TAKE PAIN MEDICATIONS?

Doctors are trained to diagnose and treat diseases and injuries and minimize suffering. Unfortunately, many doctors do not know the difference between nociceptive, neuropathic and nociplastic pain. Medical curriculum teaches about diseases that can initiate pain, such as diabetes, bone fractures, inflammatory arthritis, but they fail to teach what to do when the pain transitions from acute to chronic pain.

As we now know, drugs, injections and surgery are the best tools to treat acute pain from nociceptive or neuropathic origins, but rarely have a benefit effect on nociplastic pain. However, when physicians encounter patients with chronic pain, they generally use the tools they know best: drugs, injections and surgery. Physicians who receive more visits from pharmaceutical industry representatives tend to prescribe more drugs, as they are informed about the wonders these drugs can do for their patients. And patients go to their doctors asking for a new prescription after they see TV ads for "amazing" new drugs.

Conquering Chronic Pain without Pain Medications

When it is possible, my preference is to manage chronic pain without pain medications, or with the least amount necessary or for the shortest possible period of time.

The following are some reasons for not using medications to treat chronic pain.

- Some types of chronic pain do not respond well to pain medications.
- Opioid use can result in opioids-induced hyperalgesia, in which opioids amplify pain.
- Many drugs used to treat pain impair concentration, attention and memory.
- Various pain drugs cause problems with digestion, sleep quality, breathing, immune response, bone metabolism, skin and sex hormones.
- The body quickly develops physical dependence when pain medications are used daily.
- There is a risk of developing substance-use disorder with many pain drugs such as opioids, cannabinoids and benzodiazepines.

- Intoxication, overdose and death may occur with acetaminophen, NSAIDs, opioids, antidepressants, benzodiazepines and anticonvulsants.
- Drug-to-drug interaction is very common among pain medications and with medications used to treat other conditions.
- Strong reliance on pain medications leads to low motivation to attempt other treatments for pain, such as movement, mind-body therapies and other modalities.
- There is financial strain on the person and on the healthcare system because of the high costs of some newer medications.
- Driving a car becomes very dangerous when a person takes painkillers that affect their ability to react quickly to a dangerous situation on the road.
- Sleep becomes disrupted by medications that affect the sleep cycle, causing drowsiness during the day and tiredness.
- Absorption of nutrients from diet is essential to conquering chronic pain, but for many people their digestive system is affected with nausea, vomiting and constipation caused by pain medications.
- Some types of chronic pain do not respond well to pain medications.

However, there are situations, especially when there is an ongoing nociceptive or neuropathic pain, in which giving pain medications improves a patient's quality of life dramatically.

> Are you a person who takes lots of medications
> or someone who avoids and hates pills?
> I would love to hear which side of the fence you are on.
> Answer by tagging me on social media with
> #ConquerPainWithDrFurlan.

"Some types of chronic pain do not respond well to pain medications."

Cutting back on multiple prescriptions

It is very common for patients with chronic pain to be seen by multiple prescribers and to keep adding more and more drugs. Even when they are not sure if they are benefiting from all these prescriptions, they are reluctant to stop taking them in case their pain gets worse.

As well, many patients feel worse when they try to stop their regular medications. This can be confusing. They think they need these medications because when they try to skip a dose or stop their pain medications, they feel pain coming back. But many times, what they are feeling are withdrawal symptoms from stopping a medication to which they have developed a physical dependence.

I feel worse when I stop taking my regular medication. Is that because I am addicted to it?

Not necessarily. Physical dependence is not the same as being addicted or having a substance-use disorder. Physical dependence is necessary to develop an addiction. But you can be physically dependent on a medication and have withdrawal symptoms without having a substance-use disorder. (We talk more about addiction when we discuss opioids, but we refer to it as opioid-use disorder. See page 204.) Ask your doctor if what you are feeling is your pain "coming back" or if you are having withdrawal symptoms. Ask for help in managing your symptoms.

Physical dependence and withdrawal symptoms

Physical dependence occurs with many medications, not only opioids. It is not the same thing as addiction. Physical dependence occurs when a person takes medication regularly, daily, and the body gets used to its effects. Then, when that substance is stopped, the body shows typical symptoms called withdrawal symptoms, or abstinence syndrome.

Following is a list of substances that cause physical dependence and withdrawal symptoms.

SUBSTANCE	TYPICAL WITHDRAWAL SYMPTOMS
Alcohol	Shaky hands, headache, vomiting, sweating, agitation
Opioids	Abdominal pain, diarrhea, headache, muscle aches, agitation, anxiety
Anti-acid proton pump inhibitor (PPI)	Rebound acid hyperproduction, indigestion, heartburn, regurgitation
Blood pressure medication, propranolol	Sweating, shaking, irregular heartbeat and chest pain
Thyroid hormones	Anxiety, panic attacks, fatigue, muscle weakness, diarrhea, nausea

Rebound headaches

In the case of headaches and migraines, there are many painkillers that cause a condition called medication overuse headache. This means that the painkillers will perpetuate the pain, so that every time the person stops taking the drugs, they have rebound headaches. This happens with acetaminophen, non-steroidal anti-inflammatories (NSAIDs), ergotamine, triptans, barbiturates and opioids.

TIPS TO IMPROVE REBOUND HEADACHES

- Tell your doctor and pharmacist that you want to eliminate some headache medications. They can help by providing some prevention drugs or bridge therapy. Bridge therapy includes medications such as anti-nausea medications to reduce the withdrawal symptoms.
- For simple situations, the best approach is to stop cold turkey.
- For complex situations, as when you are taking an opioid, or have severe anxiety, you may need close supervision.

"Physical dependence occurs when a person takes medication regularly, daily, and the body gets used to its effects."

Prescription Medications for Chronic Pain

Opioids

Let me address the elephant in the room.

Opioids are powerful analgesics. Codeine and morphine are found naturally in the poppy plants. Others are made synthetically in a laboratory. All opioids are compared to morphine in terms of potency. Some are less potent than morphine, so they require a higher dose to achieve the same effects of morphine, while others are more potent than morphine, and they require a lower amount to achieve the same effects.

However, opioids have become a major point of concern in North America, with a so-called opioid crisis taking many lives in unintentional overdoses and a plethora of people who have developed opioid-use disorder. So now, prescribing opioids has become a subject of much debate.

You might be aware of the stories in the news. You worry that your body is getting accustomed to opioids. You don't feel the same pain relief that you felt the first time you tried it. It seems the pills are losing their effect and your body is getting used to them. You worry that you are becoming addicted to this drug. Your family tells you to stop taking them.

Your doctor continues prescribing and pushing you to take more pills. Or maybe your doctor is worried that you are taking too many painkillers.

What should you do?

Rather than discuss the origins and causes of the "opioid crisis," I prefer to give a balanced view of the role opioids can play in the management of chronic pain.

WATCH MY VIDEO ON OPIOID-INDUCED HYPERALGESIA

OPIOIDS ARE HELPFUL FOR ONLY A MINORITY OF CHRONIC PAIN PATIENTS

It is my opinion that opioids are helpful for a minority of patients with a well-defined nociceptive or neuropathic chronic pain condition. Pain responds well to opioids when there is an ongoing injury, lesion or illness. When the pain becomes nociplastic (when there is central sensitization), opioids do not have the same benefits. There are more effective treatments for chronic pain of nociplastic origin.

FAQ

What is opioid-induced hyperalgesia?

We know that some changes occur in the NMDA receptors and neurotransmitters when there is sensitization of the pain system. If you add opioids to these neuronal changes, it is like adding gasoline to the fire.

The resulting condition is *opioid-induced hyperalgesia* or, in other terms, pain caused by opioids.

Initially, when the patient receives the first few doses of opioids, the pain is very much reduced. They really feel better and are happy that finally someone has given them a pill that reduces pain. But as they continue taking those pills every day, the opioid will start activating those "modified NMDA receptors" in their pain system, and they will start having a condition called hyperalgesia.

Hyperalgesia has two main characteristics. First, the pain starts spreading. A pain that was confined to one small area starts affecting a larger area of the body. Second, the skin gets more sensitive to touch. Normally, when we touch the skin with a cotton ball, the person will feel a cotton ball. However, in hyperalgesia, the cotton ball feels like sandpaper rubbing their skin. If we touch the skin with a toothpick, the person feels it like a knife.

The treatment for opioid-induced hyperalgesia is slowly reducing the dose of opioid. We call this tapering. With this gradual reduction in dose, the pain system starts reverting to its original normal state.

"How can opioids make the pain worse if I feel better when I take my opioid pill"?

I commonly have patients who have trouble believing that an opioid can make their pain worse. Here are some of the things they tell me:

- "When I am feeling terrible, I take the pill and then I feel better. Obviously, this pill must be doing something good to me."
- "Doctor, please do not tell me to stop taking this pill. It is the only thing that works for me."
- "I have been taking these pills for so long, but I am not addicted, and I am not abusing. So please let me continue taking them."

HELEN AND HER NIGHT SWEATS

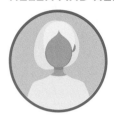 Helen was a 75-year-old woman who had suffered with chronic pain for more than 20 years. Her doctor had been prescribing her opioids and increasing the dose, but she was still in a lot of pain. When she came to me, she was taking an equivalent of 900 mg of morphine per day, which is an extremely high dosage.

She had pain in multiple parts of her body and never left her house except for medical appointments. She could not sleep at night because of profuse sweating. She had severe constipation with only one bowel movement per week. She wanted to know what else she could take to treat her pain.

I explained to her that the opioid dose was extremely high, and that her sweating and constipation were side effects of opioids. When I told her that the opioid itself could cause her pain, she was open to reducing its dose.

It took a few months to reduce the opioid dose to half. She felt much better, but was still in pain. We continued lowering the dose, and then switched her to a different opioid called buprenorphine. We had to do that because her body was very physically dependent on the opioid and it was almost impossible to stop her opioids completely. Buprenorphine is a type of opioid that causes fewer withdrawal symptoms and less physical dependence.

After that, Helen was another person. Her husband came to the follow-up appointment with her to thank our team. He told us she was much more alert, went out with friends, walked more than a mile (2 km) every day, and her constipation and sweats disappeared. Besides, she could sleep the whole night.

She stayed on the opioid buprenorphine, and she no longer needed to see us.

"Rotating from one opioid to another has many advantages."

Why would any doctor want to rock the boat of these patients? It seems so counterintuitive. Maybe even cruel and inhumane. If it is helping, why not let them have it?

The answer is simple: Are they still in pain?

If they still have pain, then the opioid might just be aggravating the pain in the background. And when the person "feels better," it is most likely they are treating withdrawal from the previous dose of opioid. We call this withdrawal mediated pain.

WITHDRAWAL SYMPTOMS

Earlier in this chapter, I explained physical dependence, and I gave you examples of drugs, including blood pressure medications and thyroid hormones, that cause physical dependence.

If your body is used to opioids, when you skip a dose, or when you are late to take your next pill, you start having withdrawal symptoms. It feels like a bad flu. Then, once you take the opioid, the withdrawal symptoms disappear, including the pain from the opioid withdrawal.

We produce our own opioids, but when we take opioids as a drug, our internal stock is reduced.

Human beings are born with *opioid receptors* because we are able to produce our own *endogenous* (internal) opioids: endorphins, enkephalins and dynorphins. But once we start taking *exogenous* (external) opioids, either in pills by mouth, transdermal patches, or injected in the muscles or intravenously, our own "factory" of endogenous opioids is reduced.

Most patients do not even remember what a life without opioids is. They have been taking opioids for so many months, or years, that their "normal" is what it feels like being under the influence of opioids. When they do not fill those opioid receptors with opioid, their body is unable to produce their own endogenous opioids, and instead they produce the very unpleasant withdrawal symptoms.

In people who have used exogenous opioids for many years, once they stop taking them, their body will need to reactivate the production of endogenous opioids. However, this may take weeks, months or even years.

I tell my patients that for each year that they have used opioids, we will need to wait about one month for their endogenous opioids to kick in again. So, a patient who had

For tips on how to talk with your doctor about either starting or stopping using opioids, see page 175–177 in *Step 5: Get Help from Others*. We explore more effective treatments for chronic pain of nociplastic origin in the next chapter, *Step 7: Make Room in Your Toolbox*.

WATCH MY VIDEO ON OPIOID TAPERING

been receiving daily opioids for 12 years, we will need to wait about 12 months until their own endogenous production ramps up.

This is why I suggest, if someone wants to stop taking opioids, they should start reducing the dose slowly, and allow time for their body to adapt to the new normal. We call this a slow tapering protocol.

> If someone wants to stop taking opioids, they should start reducing the dose slowly, and allow time for their body to adapt to the new normal.

OPIOID-USE DISORDER

Opioid-use disorder is one of the substance-use disorders we discussed in *Step 2: Control Your Emotions.* Remember, substance-use disorder is a disease and not an indication of a weak person.

Opioid-use disorder is rare among patients who use opioids for chronic pain. It is estimated that 5 percent of people who use daily opioids will develop signs and symptoms of opioid-use disorder. However, given that there are millions of people with chronic pain who are prescribed daily opioids, the number of potential people who are at risk of developing opioid-use disorder is large.

Once these patients exhibit signs of opioid-use disorder, such as craving opioids, running out early before the next refill or using more than prescribed, that is when doctors get concerned about these behaviors.

Often the response is to stop prescribing their opioids. Instead of making the diagnosis of opioid-use disorder and treating them early, the doctor does the opposite of what should be done and stops prescribing opioids.

Cutting the patient off from their opioids puts them at a high risk of anxiety, depression, despair, suicide or getting opioids from illicit sources. Many patients who resort to illicit sources end up buying opioids from questionable sources, and these can contain opioids contaminated with fentanyl. Because fentanyl is 50 to 100 times more potent than morphine, the worst, a fatal accidental overdose, can happen.

Antidepressants

Neuropathic pain leads to many changes in the pain system and these changes deplete the neurotransmitter serotonin. When serotonin is low in the brain, the person feels sad and has low energy. It is very common for those with chronic pain to also have depressive mood disorder. We use antidepressants to raise the serotonin levels in the brain.

There are cases of nociplastic pain that also improve with antidepressants, especially in people with fibromyalgia and myofascial pain syndrome. The problem is the side effects. Many patients do not tolerate the dry mouth, constipation, dizziness, tiredness and weight gain caused by antidepressants.

There are many types of antidepressants. We may try one, and if it causes too many side effects, try another one, and so on. The main types of antidepressants we use for chronic pain are tricyclic antidepressants (amitriptyline, nortriptyline) and serotonin norepinephrine reuptake inhibitors or SNRIs (duloxetine, venlafaxine and milnacipran).

We start with the lowest possible dose and increase gradually to avoid side effects. If we start with a medium or high dose, the patient usually discontinues the treatment because the side effects seem intolerable. These medications need a prescription from your doctor.

Amitriptyline and duloxetine are examples of medications I recommend most of the time. Of course, I do make changes depending on the patient's tolerance level and previous experience with antidepressants. Your doctor may suggest a different dose scheme, and that is perfectly fine. Always follow your doctor's prescription.

WATCH MY VIDEO ON AMITRIPTYLINE

WATCH MY VIDEO ON DULOXETINE

FAQ

Why do doctors prescribe antidepressants to treat chronic pain?

We prescribe antidepressant medications to treat chronic pain because they increase monoamine neurotransmitters in certain areas of the pain system. These transmitters are responsible for controlling certain biological, emotional and behavioral functions that are abnormal in people with chronic pain.

Duloxetine is an antidepressant of the serotonin-noradrenaline reuptake inhibitor (SNRI) class. We use duloxetine when the person has chronic pain, depressed mood and/or anxiety disorder. (See *Step 2: Control Your Emotions*, on page 104, for more about how antidepressants help with chronic pain.)

WHAT KIND OF BENEFITS CAN YOU EXPECT WITH ANTIDEPRESSANTS?

- The first benefit you will notice when you take antidepressants is in your sleep. It will knock you down. This can be noticeable right away. But it is important to keep working on your sleep quality, as we discussed in *Step 3: Get Quality Sleep.* We don't want to use antidepressants for a long time, as they disrupt some sleep architecture. So, when we start weaning the antidepressants, you should already be practicing the strategies mentioned in *Step 3.*
- A few weeks after you start an antidepressant, you will notice some reduction in pain intensity. Because the drug needs time to build up serotonin in the brain, a patient needs to take them daily for a couple of weeks to obtain pain relief.
- The last benefit you will notice, maybe a couple of weeks or month after you start, is in your mood.

WATCH MY VIDEO ON GABAPENTIN

Antiepileptics

Antiepileptic drugs, also known as anticonvulsants, are used to treat chronic pain because they stop the firing from the neurons and therefore, they reduce the brain activity.

They are useful for cases of neuropathic pain such as post-stroke, spinal cord injury, multiple sclerosis and nerve injuries. They have been used in patients with central sensitization caused by nociplastic pain, but the results are not too exciting.

There are a couple of different antiepileptic drugs that can be used for pain. Gabapentin and pregabalin are very similar in their formula, indications and side effects. Pregabalin is more potent than gabapentin, so the doses are lower and it can be taken twice a day, instead of three times a day for gabapentin.

WATCH MY VIDEO ON PREGABALIN

We usually start at the lowest possible dose to avoid intolerable side effects.

Muscle relaxants

Muscle relaxants do not act in the muscles; they act in the brain, which controls the muscles. They can be obtained without a prescription in most pharmacies, although in some countries they are controlled medications and need a doctor's prescription. This group includes drugs such as methocarbamol, orphenadrine and chlorzoxazone. Their main adverse effect is causing sedation, and therefore they need to be taken with caution by people who drive or operate heavy machinery at work.

There is another class of muscle relaxants that are used when the muscles have spasticity, which is a rigidity of the muscles caused by neurological conditions such as cerebral palsy, stroke, spinal cord injury and multiple sclerosis. This group of medications include baclofen, dantrolene and tizanidine.

Finally, benzodiazepines, which are medications used for anxiety and insomnia, can also be used as muscle relaxants, but only for a short period, as they produce tolerance and physical dependence very quickly.

> Muscle relaxants do not act in the muscles, they act in the brain, which controls the muscles.

WATCH MY VIDEO ON MUSCLE RELAXANTS

Medications applied by injections

BOTULINUM TOXIN

Botulinum toxin has been used for decades to reduce muscle tone in people with spasticity, as seen in cerebral palsy, stroke and spinal cord injury. More recently, it has been used to treat painful conditions without spasticity, such as chronic low back pain, cervical dystonia (involuntary neck spasms), lazy eye, overactive bladder, hyperhidrosis (abnormal sweating) and chronic migraines.

This medication is derived from a toxin produced by bacteria and it blocks the muscle contractions temporarily. The toxin can be found in some types of food poisoning and can lead to death by muscle paralysis, a condition called botulism.

The injections must be applied by a trained medical professional at specific sites in the muscles. The muscles will become weaker until the nerve regrows and that muscle becomes stronger again, which process takes about three months.

KETAMINE

Ketamine is an anesthetic agent used in general anesthesia. In lower doses it has been used to treat psychiatric disorders, including major depressive disorder and neuropathic pain.

There are risks to using ketamine. For this reason, it must be carefully used under supervision and for a specific objective. It can lead to dissociative symptoms and should be avoided in people with psychotic disorders. It is highly addictive, so it should be avoided in people with an active substance-use disorder.

LIDOCAINE AND NERVE BLOCKS

Lidocaine is a type of local anesthetic. It blocks the electrical impulses in the nerves and is helpful for surgical procedures that do not require general anesthesia. The block is temporary and lasts a couple of hours. The anesthetized area becomes numb and the surgeon can perform the procedure.

Local anesthetics are also used to do diagnostic nerve blocks. These are targeted injections, usually done under ultrasound or fluoroscopic imaging (basically, real-time, moving X-rays). The anesthetist blocks a specific nerve that is thought to be the pain generator. In some cases of chronic pain, it may be caused by nerve compression or a localized injury. If the chronic pain is greatly relieved after a nerve block, then the physician may suggest performing a permanent block of that nerve, by destroying or removing that part of the nerve.

Lidodaine is also used for trigger point injections. These are tight and painful spots in the muscles that feel like knots. These trigger points irradiate pain to large areas away from the painful spots. Trigger point injections will block the pain and also provide mechanical stimulation that will increase blood circulation and bring more oxygen to the area, therefore breaking the pain cycle.

SYMPATHETIC BLOCKS

There are some conditions that involve the sympathetic nervous system, such as complex regional pain syndrome (CRPS), Raynaud's disease and cluster headaches. A sympathetic block involves an injection of a local anesthetic to block the activity of the sympathetic nervous system to that area of the body. The sympathetic nervous system controls the veins, arteries, sweating glands, skin temperature and many other functions in our body that are controlled by the autonomous nerve system.

CORTICOSTEROID INJECTIONS

Cortisone is a type of steroid. It can be administered to the body by mouth, inhalers, intranasal sprays, eye drops, topical creams or injections.

A cortisone injection is used to reduce inflammation, and it is commonly injected inside the inflamed joints or around a tendon. There is a maximum limit of how many cortisone injections one can get in each joint, as too many will accelerate the destruction of the cartilage and lead to osteoarthritis. The effect of steroid injections in the joint lasts months, as this is how long the deposits of steroid take to be reabsorbed by the circulatory system. Cortisone shots can be given to any joint in the body, including the temporomandibular joint, spine, shoulders, elbows, wrists, hands, hips, knees, ankles and feet.

WATCH MY VIDEO ON CORTISONE INJECTIONS

TOPICAL CREAMS

Many drugs are absorbed by the skin. There are some ready-made ointments, creams and lotions that contain medicinal ingredients for pain, muscle relaxation and inflammation. In other cases, we need to prescribe a special compounded cream that is individualized to each patient.

The choice to use topical creams depends on the size of the area that has pain, and if the origin of the pain is localized. For example, if the pain is from a small inflammatory arthritis of the hand, a topical cream containing anti-inflammatories could be used, instead of taking tablets by mouth. Another example would be a herpes zoster affecting a small area of the skin. Instead of using neuropathic pain pills or tablets, a topical cream could cover the area and provide relief.

Medications for Chronic Pain that Do Not Need a Doctor's Prescription

There are pain relief medications that do not need a physician's prescription. They are found in pharmacies and are classified as over-the-counter (OTC) or behind-the-counter (BTC) medications. OTC medicines can be found on the shelves and do not need authorization from the pharmacist. BTC medications are not found on the shelves because they need to be authorized by the pharmacist.

For information on magnesium and other dietary supplements that may to help relieve your pain, see *Step 4: Fix Your Diet,* pages 150–156.

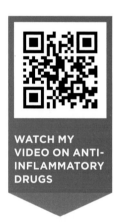

WATCH MY VIDEO ON ANTI-INFLAMMATORY DRUGS

There is a perception that OTC medications are safe because they do not require a physician's prescription. This is false. People can abuse and die of intoxication of these medications.

OTC medications can cause serious adverse events if the dosage and delivery instructions enclosed or printed on the container are not followed properly. Always read this information.

- *Acetaminophen* can cause acute liver failure if the dose exceeds 3,000 mg in a day. Many people do not know that there are cough syrups, headache medications and flu medications that contain acetaminophen. And when all of those are added together, it is not hard to take a high dose. In North America, many people suffer from liver failure and are waiting for a liver transplant because of too much acetaminophen.
- *Acetylsalicylic acid,* branded as Aspirin, should not be given to children under 18 years of age with fever, as this may cause Reye's syndrome, a life-threatening condition.
- *Anti-inflammatories like ibuprofen or naproxen* may increase the risk of a heart attack and stroke in a person with existing heart problems.
- *Diclofenac and misoprostol* should not be given to pregnant women, as they may cause serious bleeding and premature birth.

Cannabinoids

Our body has receptors for cannabinoids because we produce our own cannabinoids. These receptors are distributed in various organs and tissues of the body. One of our endogenous (internal) cannabinoids is called anandamide.

The cannabis plant has more than 500 substances. Of those, at least 113 are cannabinoids, which have an effect on the human body's receptors CB1 and CB2.

There are synthetic cannabinoids made in the laboratory, such as dronabinol and nabilone. Nabilone is approved in Canada and it is available for severe nausea and vomiting from cancer chemotherapy. It can be used for AIDS-related anorexia, palliative pain and neuropathic pain.

The two most studied cannabinoids from the cannabis plant are tetrahydrocannabinol (THC) and cannabidiol (CBD). Some cannabis plants will not produce THC or CBD, but others will produce one or the other. The effects of THC are mainly in the brain. It causes euphoria and relaxation. CBD does not cause euphoria and therefore it is not used for recreational purposes, but it does cause sleepiness.

Cannabinoids from cannabis have been used in medicine mainly for the treatment of some conditions such as chemotherapy-induced nausea and vomiting, spasticity related to multiple sclerosis, seizures and severe neuropathic pain. However, there are not a lot of scientific studies demonstrating how CBD acts to relieve pain.

What are the benefits of using cannabinoids for chronic pain?

- There is some evidence that THC improves neuropathic pain.
- CBD seems to be beneficial for chronic pain, and it does not cause euphoria. However, it causes drowsiness and sleepiness.
- Some patients have been able to stop using their opioids because they started using cannabinoids, either synthetic or from the cannabis plant.
- There are no reports of people who have died of overdose or intoxication due to cannabis, which is not the case for opioids, which may cause overdose and death.
- There is some anecdotal evidence that THC and CBD help with sleep and anxiety.
- Using oils that contain extracts from the plant is better than smoking cannabis. A licensed producer will grow the plant and extract only the cannabinoids that are medically indicated, either THC or CBD or both, removing all other unwanted substances from the oils.

WATCH MY VIDEO ON CANNABINOIDS

Nicotine products

One in five people with chronic pain smokes.

Most people don't know that smoking cigarettes predisposes a person to chronic pain, such as low back pain, rheumatoid arthritis, headaches and neuropathic pain.

Some people say they smoke because of their pain. They endorse smoking as a pain-coping mechanism, a distraction.

However, most people also don't know that nicotine has analgesic properties, which means it is a painkiller. In human volunteer studies, people reported less intense pain when they were given nicotine before the experiment to provoke pain. The response occurs mainly at the brain level when the nicotine activates receptors that result in the release of opioid and norepinephrine in the brain (Shi, 2010). This blocks the bottom-up pain activating pathways and will stimulate the top-down pain inhibitory pathways in the pain system. (See pages 22–25 in *What Is Pain?*) In other words, nicotine can decrease pain. But because it creates physical dependence, nicotine is not a good analgesic.

Some people keep smoking because they don't want to gain weight if they quit. However, the weight gain is between 2 and 5 pounds (1–2.3 kg), and the health benefits of quitting are much greater than the risk of gaining just 5 pounds.

Various mechanisms explain why people who smoke have more chronic pain. There are more than 4,000 substances in a cigarette, and when people smoke every day, these substances will:

- Damage many body tissues and organs with impaired bone healing, wound healing, osteoporosis and disk disease. The carbon monoxide will lead to poor oxygenation of organs.
- Upset the pain system and lead to nociplastic pain
- Interact with opioids, causing cross-tolerance and altered breakdown of opioids
- Alter mood. People who smoke are more depressed. Nicotine increases the hormone norepinephrine, which increases blood pressure and affects mood and anxiety.
- Lead to nicotine dependence. Nicotine will reach the brain within a few seconds after the first inhalation, then release dopamine, which is the neurotransmitter of pleasure and reward. Nicotine withdrawal symptoms are very severe.

I know many orthopedic surgeons who will not operate on someone who smokes cigarettes. That is because smoking impairs oxygen delivery to tissues, including bones, impairing bone healing and wound healing, and could contribute to complications such as infections, poor healing and pain after surgery.

"Many orthopedic surgeons will not operate on someone who smoke cigarettes."

Your medication concerns and goals

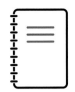

Let's do another exercise. Do you worry about your medication? Now that you have more information, do you have any new thoughts or concerns about your medication?

The following are some of the common concerns that I hear from my patients.

- "Will I be able to reduce the number of medications I take?"
- "I wish I didn't need one medication for pain and then many others for the side effects caused by the painkiller. Can the dose of some medications be decreased?"
- "Can I travel abroad without worrying if my prescriptions will be filled at the pharmacies in another country?"
- "Can I drive my car or operate heavy machinery at work without being worried that my attention and motor control are putting me or my coworkers at risk of an accident?"
- "If I didn't take so many pills, I wouldn't have to worry about my liver, kidney and stomach being damaged by them."
- "Maybe I don't need to be concerned anymore about overdosing and getting addicted to these pills."
- "I don't want to worry about getting pregnant or breastfeeding my newborn because I am taking these pills."
- "I feel like a hostage to my doctor. I want freedom from painkillers."
- "I fear that if I lose my job I will not have health benefits and will not be able to afford these medications."
- "I lost my sex drive and the relationship with my partner is in danger."
- "When I need to see a new doctor, they ask me the medications I take, and when I say the names of the drugs I take, they look at me with that judgment face."
- "My pharmacist keeps telling me I need to stop these medications. I hate when I have to go to the pharmacy to get my prescriptions."

❶ Now, take out your journal and record your own concerns about your medication. Include any goals you may have. If there is anything you want to discuss with your pain medication team, write it down.

FRED AND A SUCCESSFUL POLYPHARMACY

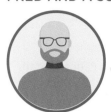

Fred was 54 years of age when he had a thalamic stroke. The thalamus is the part of the brain that functions as the relay of all sensations from the body. A stroke in the thalamus can cause very serious sensory problems, including a type of neuropathic pain known as central post-stroke pain. This is one of the worst kinds of pain known to humankind. Some patients describe it as a hot oil burning all the time on the part affected by the stroke.

To treat Fred's pain we had to try various medications, from various different classes. This type of pain is very resistant to all kinds of treatments, but we persisted and tried various drugs. We ended up finding a combination of three medications that give him about 70 percent pain relief. They include an opioid, an anticonvulsant and a cannabinoid called nabilone.

He is able to return to work full time and enjoy his family and friends.

This case illustrates that sometimes it takes many months, or years, to arrive at a combination of medications (we call this polypharmacy) that works for a patient.

We need to change one drug at a time, and wait until we reach a reasonable dose of that drug, then we let the drug stablilize for a few weeks or months and we reevaluate. If the doctor or the patient gives up too early, they may lose the opportunity to find just the right combination for that person. And each person is different, so we need to individualize the treatment.

"To find out if a drug is helpful for chronic pain, we need to increase the dose slowly until we reach a proper dose and stabilize it. This may take many weeks to a couple of months."

CONCLUSION

There is freedom on the other side of the mountain. It is possible to reduce your use of pain medications. Now that you have read this chapter, you have more information on your side. You can discuss your medications with your nurse, pharmacist and your doctor.

KEY POINTS TO REMEMBER

- If you take medications for pain, you need to understand why you take each of them and what they do to your body. Also, you need to be sure you really need them.
- Painkillers are designed to reduce pain intensity. The most common are acetaminophen, anti-inflammatories and opioids. These medications are not free from side effects and complications.
- When in doubt, consult your pharmacist, nurse or your doctor. They can answer most of your questions and address your concerns.
- If your pain medications are not reducing the pain intensity and improving your function by at least 30 percent, they may not be helping you at all.
- Not everyone with chronic pain needs to take medication. It is possible to control pain without medications.
- Opioids are useful for acute pain after an injury, surgery or for treatment of cancer-related pain. Their prolonged use in chronic pain may make the pain worse, impair concentration and attention and cause side effects. More rarely, opioid use could lead to overdose, addiction and death.
- Some antidepressants and anticonvulsants are used to treat neuropathic pain.
- Some medications can be applied by injection or topical creams.

LOOKING AHEAD

In the next chapter, *Step 7: Make Room in Your Toolbox*, we discuss other options to manage pain, including therapeutic movement, manual therapies, massage, alternative and complementary medicine as well as heat, cold and electrotherapy.

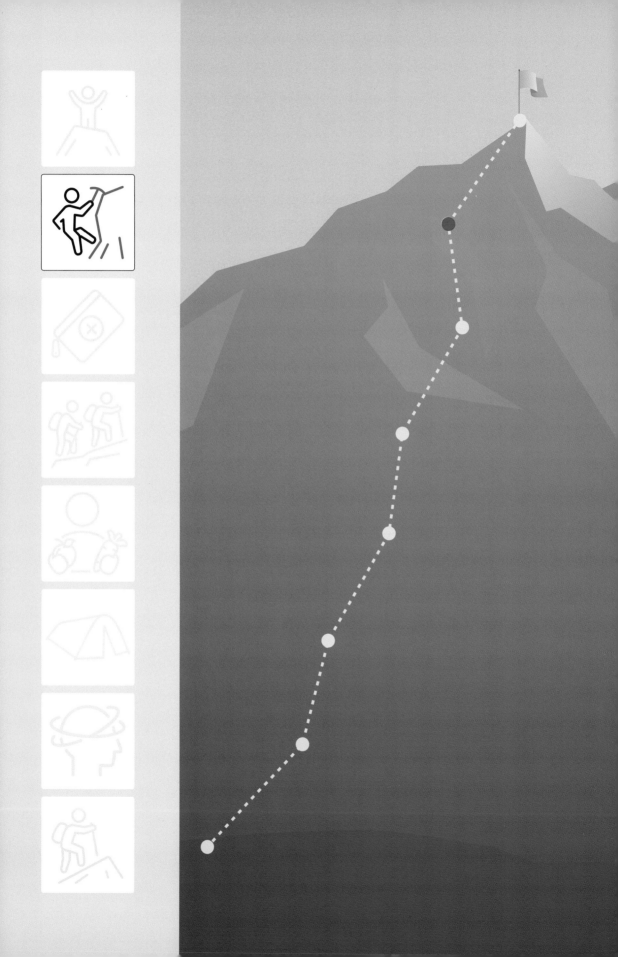

Make Room in Your Toolbox

So far, the mountaineer has survived the storm, the cold nights, the blazing sunlight, the dehydration, the lack of oxygen and the muscle cramps. At this point, they feel they can handle any situation. The group is composed of novice and experienced mountaineers, so they gather at night to share their experiences and learn from each other. They share strategies. For each situation, there is a solution. For each challenge, a way to break through. For simple problems, they found a quick fix. For complex conditions, they took an analytical and systematic approach to the climb. They didn't restrict themselves to just one way of meeting the challenges.

We've looked at how you can learn to retrain your mind and control your emotions in your journey to conquer chronic pain. We've considered how you can best communicate with others about your pain. And we've looked at the various medications that can help you manage your pain. But drugs aren't the only tools you need. When you are dealing with chronic pain, drugs are only one of the tools in our toolbox. There should be lots of other options in your toolbox.

In this chapter, we discuss other options to manage pain and deal with flare-ups, in particular, three of the 5Ms:

- *Movement* as a therapeutic intervention to treat chronic pain and fix the pain system
- *Manual therapies,* including massage, alternative and complementary medicine
- *Modalities* such as heat, cold and electrotherapy

We'll also look at some more suggestions for managing pain with *mind-body therapies*.

Prepare Yourself

Problem-solving requires some planning. It is hard to think of solutions when you are in the middle of a crisis. Having a flare-up of your pain can interrupt your plans, your routine and your happiness. If you anticipate a flare-up and prepare yourself for it, you will find creative solutions, less stress and more enjoyment. I have helped many people prepare a contingency plan for a bad day.

Let's go shopping for tools to put in your toolbox!

What are the tools in your toolbox?

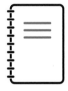

Let's do an exercise.

1. Read the case study on the facing page. Think about the tools that Sam uses to cope with his spinal stenosis. He has a long list of strategies:

☑ Exercise classes

☑ Pain-relief positions

☑ Cognitive behavioral therapy

☑ Chair cycle

☑ Meditation, prayers

☑ Hot pack

☑ Pillows

☑ Driving, helping others (distraction)

☑ Playing bocce ball

☑ Bending forward

☑ Travel (planning and enjoying)

☑ Going to restaurants

☑ Pain medication

2. How many tools do you have? Can you list at least 10 strategies that you use to cope with your pain? Get out your journal and record them.

SAM HAS A FULL TOOLBOX

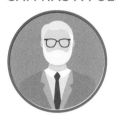 Sam is a 64-year-old male who likes to play soccer and enjoys exotic dishes at out-of-the-ordinary restaurants. His goal was to retire and travel with his wife. But his plans had to change when a problem in his lower spine required surgery. The surgery saved his bowels and bladder from becoming incontinent, but he developed chronic lower back pain that makes walking very painful. He has severe spinal stenosis, which is a problem of a narrow spinal canal compressing the spinal cord and the nerves that go to his pelvis and legs. It limits his ability to stand and walk. He doesn't feel any pain if he sits and rests, but as soon as he gets up and walks, his pain immediately becomes a 10 out of 10.

He doesn't take any medications; when he did try them, they did not help him and they caused drowsiness and balance problems.

Sam learned everything he could about spinal stenosis. He attended group exercise classes and learned positions that could alleviate his pain. He participated in cognitive behavioral therapy and incorporated pacing, mindfulness and relaxation in his routine. He bought a chair cycle to keep his legs fit and strong. He does daily meditations and prayers. He applies a hot pack at night and uses pillows to position his legs so he can sleep well on his side.

During the day, he drives around the city delivering "Meals on Wheels" to vulnerable seniors and people with disabilities. He plays bocce ball instead of soccer. He finds that bending forward improves his pain. When he is delivering food to the shelters and seniors who live alone, he feels pain, but he doesn't have time to be bothered by it, because he is busy and occupied with other peoples' problems, not his own problems.

Sam is planning to go on a trip with his wife and has selected the most exotic restaurants. He thinks he will need limited painkillers to be able to walk from the airport to the hotel and around the city, but believes that his pain will not stop him from fulfilling his retirement dream. He said when he is planning and making travel arrangements, he doesn't even pay attention to the pain.

Sam has learned what works for him.

The 5Ms: Five Different Types of Tools You Can Use

The 5Ms are strategies that you can use to manage your pain and reduce flare-ups.

In *Getting a Diagnosis,* I gave you a preview of the types of tools, or strategies, you will want to consider for managing your pain. See the chart *Seven Types of Tools to Treat Pain: 5M IS* on page 58. Two of these (I for Interventional pain management and S for Surgical procedures) are not tools you can pick up and use for yourself. You need professional help for those. But the others you can use for yourself.

To make it easier to remember, the five other strategies are grouped into five types of tools that start with the letter M. Once you learn them, you may need to buy some simple equipment, but you will be able to use them any time.

I once met a young woman who had had chronic pain since she was a teenager. She counted 102 strategies in her toolbox. She said she doesn't have a toolbox, but a full-size garage full of tools.

Not everyone needs 100 tools in their toolbox. I find that it is useful to have at least one tool from each of the five groups.

I know some people who would list 20 tools, but all from the same group. For example, they might say they use anti-inflammatories, muscle relaxants, anxiolytics, sleeping pills, antidepressants, anticonvulsants, cannabinoids, topical creams and opioids. But these are all from the "Medications" group.

You should try to get your tools from different groups. They are used differently and they complement each other, especially in case of a flare-up.

5Ms

M	Mind-body therapies
M	Movement
M	Modalities
M	Manual therapies
M	Medications

A flare-up is an acute painful episode or severe worsening of symptoms that can last anywhere from a few hours to a couple of weeks.

I would love to hear how many tools you have. Use this hashtag and tag me on social media with #ConquerPainWithDrFurlan.

MONICA AND HER HYPERMOBILITY

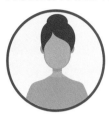 Monica is a 25-year-old female who has a condition called Ehlers-Danlos Syndrome. This is a genetic disease of the collagen tissue, which is the glue, or tape, that connects all the bones and organs to keep everything in place. Because of this condition, she has hypermobility of the joints and episodes of joint dislocations. Her joint falls out of place and needs to be put back. When this happens, she has excruciating pain, and the pain lasts a few days, even after the joint has been repositioned. These acute painful episodes are flare-ups.

She also has fibromyalgia, which makes her whole body painful all the time. Yet she says her fibromyalgia is tolerable and that she needs pain relief only when she has a flare-up.

She uses the 5M concept to remember strategies that work for her acute pain. She doesn't use them all at the same time. But she says it is good to have a list of things that work for her. Otherwise, she says, in the moment of despair, she would only remember one tool: the bottle of opioids.

Now, before reaching for her opioids, Monica tries the other Ms. They work for her and only rarely does the feel the need to take one tablet of opioid for flare-up pain.

Mind-Body Strategies

We have already explored some mind-body strategies in *Step 1: Retrain Your Pain System*, and *Step 2: Control Your Emotions*. I made these the first steps because they are the most important and most rewarding strategies you can choose to conquer chronic pain. A patient who understands how the mind and body are connected is someone who will climb their mountain and will teach others how to climb theirs.

> **Mind-body control is essential in chronic pain. We can never totally separate the mind from the body.**

In pain medicine, we use the **bio-psycho-social-spiritual model** to help the individual as a whole. That is why we recommend an interprofessional team to assess and treat individuals with chronic pain.

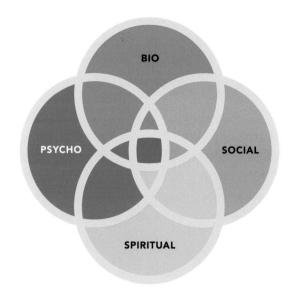

WATCH MY VIDEO ON MIND-BODY THERAPIES

The World Health Organization defines "health" as a state of complete physical, mental and social well-being and not merely the absence of disease or infirmity.

Some professions, especially doctors and pharmacists, will focus on the biological aspects of your pain.

The physiotherapist may work with your fear of movement, which is a very common psychological challenge for people with chronic pain. The nurse may work with you on increasing your knowledge about the disease and your resources to handle the symptoms. The social worker may help you to increase your social support and return to work. And a spiritual mentor may reconnect you with a faith-based group and help you to find purpose and meaning in your suffering.

In addition to the strategies we reviewed in *Step 1: Retrain Your Pain System* and *Step 2: Control Your Emotions*, following are some easy ways you can work on your mind-body connections. These strategies will help to activate the parasympathetic nervous system, reduce muscle tension and improve sleep and your mood.

A person who does not see the connection between mind and body is usually fixated on the body. They are constantly looking for a quick fix, the magic pill, the other doctor who will discover what is wrong with their body or order the diagnostic test that has not yet been done. These patients are the ones who do not get better.

MORE STRATEGIES TO HEAL MIND-BODY CONNECTIONS

ARE YOU?	WHAT IS GOING ON?	WHAT CAN YOU DO?
Afraid?	You are afraid of moving your body and causing harm. Are you afraid this is a sign of something serious and no doctor seems to know what is going on? Are you afraid your pain is getting worse and you will not be able to tolerate it anymore? **This is a fear-avoidance behavior.**	Read a book, listen to an audiobook, watch videos or talk to a counselor or therapist about CBT techniques to help you see the connections between your thoughts and emotions and between your emotions and your behaviors. Start an exercise routine. Join a gym or virtual classes.
A worrier?	You worry about your health, your body, your appearance, your reputation, your performance, your finances and your relationships. Do you wake up in the middle of the night worrying? **This is anxiety.**	Practice relaxation, meditation and mindfulness. Listen to soft and relaxing music. Learn a new skill that combines mind and movement, such as singing, dancing or sports. Pay less attention to the news. Spend less time on social media.
A perfectionist?	Are you constantly pointing out the defects, the problems and imperfections in your life and others' peoples' lives? Do you procrastinate a lot? Do you have many unfinished projects? This is a good personality trait to have, as it can get you good grades in school and high-paid jobs. But it comes with a price — your own health. **This is fear of failure.**	Practice gratitude. Be thankful for the material stuff you already have. Be grateful for the body you have. Make a list of your achievements of the past week, past month or past year. Volunteer hours to help a local charity or do something for other people. Celebrate occasions and important dates. Widen your circle of friends who support and admire you.
A people pleaser?	Are you saying yes to everyone and doing all the work? Do you have difficulty saying no because they may not like you? Are you afraid of saying no and missing a significant opportunity or promotion? **This is burnout and fear of rejection.**	Practice self-compassion. Take time for yourself. Schedule fun time in your agenda. Schedule vacation and local trips. Start a new hobby. Play with your pets or get a new pet if you like them.

ARE YOU?	WHAT IS GOING ON?	WHAT CAN YOU DO?
A victim?	You feel that your problems are the consequence of injustices and mistreatment. You blame others for your pain. You have a difficult time forgiving and forgetting what they did to you. **This is perceived injustice.**	Speak to a counselor or a spiritual guide. Practice forgiveness. Read a book, listen to an audiobook or watch videos about forgiveness. Learn the benefits to your mental and physical health when you let go of past injustices.
A pessimist?	You are certain that if something can go wrong it will. You cannot believe that something will end up going well. The only possible outcome is a tragedy and more pain. **This is catastrophizing.**	Look back in time and remember the occasions when you thought things would go badly and they actually ended up well. Talk to a counselor or mental health specialist about CBT or other techniques to help you overcome your tendency to think the worst will happen.

Movement-Based Strategies

The human body is made to move. It has bones, muscles, joints, tendons and ligaments, all connected to enable us to go from place to place.

Our society has shifted in the past 100 years and we rely more on escalators, elevators and automobiles. At home, we use a clothes washer, dishwasher, electric vacuum, lawnmower, snow blower and more to do work we used to do by moving. Then we pay for membership at a gym that we rarely find time to attend.

The comfort of a sedentary life come with a price. The less we move our body, the higher the incidence of:

- Osteoarthritis
- Osteoporosis
- Muscle tension
- Depression
- Insomnia
- Obesity
- Diabetes
- High blood pressure
- High cholesterol

Not surprisingly, the more we move our bodies, the less likely we are to experience these problems.

When I tell my patients they need to exercise, they often think I am talking about physiotherapy. Although physiotherapy usually includes movement-based therapy, some physiotherapists apply only passive modalities to reduce the pain.

Benefits of movement

There are so many benefits of movement, and not just for pain. Movement:

- Increases the production of endorphins, our natural opioids, which reduces pain
- Lubricates the joints, reducing the progression of osteoarthritis and improving stiffness and range of motion
- Prevents dementia and cognitive decline
- Increases blood flow to the brain, therefore increasing creativity and memory
- Improves blood circulation, decreases the risks of blood clots, stroke/myocardial infarct, and reduces blood pressure
- Increases lung capacity to oxygenate the blood
- Reduces risks of developing cancer
- Stimulates the immune cells, reducing the risks of infections
- Lowers cholesterol and unhealthy fat accumulation, therefore decreasing fatty liver disease, atherosclerosis, hypertension, obesity and metabolic syndrome
- Improves digestion, reduces constipation and bloating
- Improves mood, reduces stress and reduces symptoms of depression and anxiety
- Improves self-esteem, posture, confidence and energy
- Improves sleep quality and efficiency
- Prevents osteoporosis, improves balance, reduces risks of falls and fractures
- Reduces blood sugars and helps to control diabetes

> Movement increases the production of endorphins, the feel-good neuro-transmitters.

The FITT Principle

The FITT Principle (ACSM, 2022) can guide you in your decisions about how to start an exercise routine. FITT stands for Frequency, Intensity, Time and Type.

If you have a physiotherapist, an occupational therapist or a personal trainer, they have probably helped you to decide these details of your exercise routine. Some patients are on their own; either they do not have access to a professional specializing in exercises, or they can't afford one.

TYPE of exercise is whatever you choose to do. I recommend you select a type of exercise that you enjoy. There is no point in starting an activity that you have always hated or don't have the aptitude to do well. There are so many types of exercises to choose from. Some you can do at home without

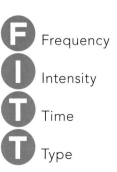

F Frequency

I Intensity

T Time

T Type

any equipment, others require some equipment and for others you need to go to a gym or a recreation center. Some people prefer to do their exercises at home, so they can do them anytime, but others like the socialization of seeing other people taking part with them.

It doesn't matter which type of exercise you do. These are some suggestions:

- **At home, without equipment:** walking indoors, stairs exercises, dancing, stretching, jumping, yoga, squats, strengthening, relaxation, square breathing
- **At home, with equipment:** treadmill, stationary bike, steps, jumping rope, weight-lifting, exercise balls, elastic bands, mats, foam rollers
- **At the gym:** treadmill, stationary bike, swimming, elliptical, rowing, weight-lifting
- **At a recreation center:** running, playing team sports, dance classes, workout classes, aqua fitness

FREQUENCY refers to how many times you plan to do these activities in a week. You may alternate days to do different activities. For example, you can go to a Zumba class once a week and do stretching at home twice a week. That is already three times a week.

INTENSITY refers to how intensely you want to exercise in each session. If you go on a treadmill, you may start at low intensity and gradually increase the speed and inclination. If you go to the gym to use the machines and gain muscle mass, you may start with the lowest weights and increase gradually.

TIME refers to how long you will perform each activity. If you have been sedentary for too long, it might be advisable to start with 15 minutes each session and gradually increase to about an hour. Ideally, you should aim for a minimum of 150 minutes of exercise every week.

THE FITT PRINCIPLES APPLIED TO FIBROMYALGIA

Exercise is an important tool in the toolbox for people with fibromyalgia. There is evidence that the benefits of exercise for fibromyalgia are greater than for than any other therapy, including medication. In the American College of Sports Medicine's *Guidelines for Exercise Testing and Prescription*, 11th Edition (ACSM, 2021]), they recommend applying the FITT principle as follows.

"Movement" is more comprehensive than "exercise" because it includes any physical activity, even the activities you do at work, going to and from work, shopping, playing with your kids, hanging your laundry on the clothesline or doing the dishes.

Aerobics exercises

FREQUENCY: Start with one to two days a week and gradually progress to two or three days a week.

INTENSITY: Begin with a light exercise and gradually progress to moderate intensity.

TIME: Start with 10 minutes a day and increase gradually to 30 to 60 minutes a day as soon as you can tolerate it.

TYPE: Enjoy low-impact exercises, such as aquatic exercise, walking, dance and other aerobic movement to music, swimming and cycling.

Resistance or strengthening exercises

FREQUENCY: Start with two to three days a week with at least 48 hours between sessions.

INTENSITY: Start with 40 to 80 percent, one repetition maximum. Gradually increase to 50 to 80 percent, one repetition maximum for strength. For muscle endurance, use 50 percent or less, one repetition maximum.

TIME: For strength, gradually progress as tolerated, increasing from 4 to 12 repetitions and from 1 to 4 sets per muscle group, with at least 2 to 3 minutes between sets. For endurance, do 15 to 20 repetitions, increasing from 1 to 2 sets with a shorter rest interval.

TYPE: You can use your own body weight, elastic bands, dumbbells, cuff/ankle weights and weight machines. For resistance exercises in water, devices can be used to create turbulence.

Flexibility or stretching

FREQUENCY: Start with two to three days a week.

INTENSITY: Stretch within limits of pain to the point of tightness or slight discomfort.

TIME: Hold each stretch for 10 to 30 seconds.

TYPE: Do static stretches (passive and/or active) for all major muscle tendon groups. You can also do dynamic stretches.

When applying these principles, people with fibromyalgia need to remember:

- You need a personalized plan. Find personal trainer who understands fibromyalgia and ask them to demonstrate the proper techniques to avoid injury.

> You need a personalized plan.

- Shorter duration sessions of four to six days a week are better than long sessions one or two days a week.
- Start low and go slow.
- Increase or decrease the intensity of these exercises depending on your perceived exertion. Go harder when you can and back off when you need to because of symptom flares.
- Pay attention to recovery time. In the beginning you may need more time between the sessions.
- If possible, choose aqua therapy exercises that include aerobics, resistance and flexibility.
- Ideal water temperature is between 91 and 97°F (33 to 36°C).
- Practice these exercises at a time of the day that is better for your symptoms.
- Do not stop these exercises during a flare-up; you may need to reduce the frequency and intensity for a short period.
- Include some stretching, breathing and relaxation techniques at the end of each session.
- Sign up for a group program for encouragement and accountability.

WATCH MY VIDEO ON FIBROMYALGIA EXERCISES

SAS EXERCISES FOR FIBROMYALGIA

S	Strengthening or resistance exercises. Weight training
A	Aerobics or cardio exercises. Accelerate the heart rate and respiratory rate
S	Stretching or flexibility exercises

Balance exercises

If you have stairs at home, then you have a great gym. How many times do you go up and down stairs every day? Did you know that you can use your staircase to do cardio, balance, strengthening and stretching exercises?

Exercises for osteoporosis

We discussed osteoporosis, the "silent thief," in *Step 4: Fix Your Diet,* on pages 150–151.

Weight-bearing exercises are essential for people who tend to develop osteoporosis. I recommend the following routine of 26 exercises that people with osteoporosis can do at home.

WATCH MY VIDEO ON BALANCE AND STRENGTH EXERCISES FOR SENIORS

THE BASE EXERCISES

These are known as the BASE exercises: Balance, Aerobics, Strengthening and Endurance.

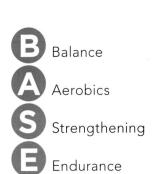

B Balance
A Aerobics
S Strengthening
E Endurance

Chair

1. Holding on to a chair, stand in place and raise heels up and down.
2. Holding on to a chair, stand on one foot, then the other foot.

Walk

3. Walk at a normal pace.
4. Walk in a straight line, one foot in front of the other, heel touching the toe.
5. Walk backwards.
6. Walk sideways.
7. Walk doing lunges.
8. Walk on your tiptoes and come back on your heels.

Bags of beans in each hand (or use wrist weights)

9. Walk at a normal pace with bags of beans.
10. Walk in tandem with bags of beans.
11. Walk backwards with bags of beans.
12. Walk sideways with bags of beans.
13. Walk doing lunges with bags of beans.
14. Walk on your tiptoes and come back on your heels with bags of beans.

Step or stairs

15. *One step:* Left foot up first, left foot down first
16. *One step:* Right foot up first, right foot down first
17. Stairs up on left foot first. Stairs down on left foot first
18. Stairs up on right foot first. Stairs down on right foot first

Chair

19. Sit to stand.
20. Sit to stand holding bags of beans
21. *If you have a resistance band:*
    a. Pull band to both sides.
    b. Place around your back, pull in front of you.
    c. Place under your thighs, pull up and down.

On the wall

22. Pushups; maintain straight spine
23. Back to the wall, posture straight, squat

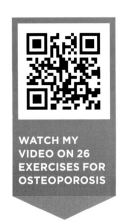

WATCH MY VIDEO ON 26 EXERCISES FOR OSTEOPOROSIS

On the wall with bags of beans

24. Back to the wall, holding bags of beans and bending the knees, slowly go down, maintain this position, move arms up and down.

25. Wall angel, holding bags of beans

On the wall

26. Fingers walking on the wall

Exercises for osteoarthritis

Osteoarthritis is a condition caused by loss of cartilage that protects the bones, reduced joint space and loss of lubricant fluid between the bones.

Over the past 20 years, scientists have discovered that osteoarthritis is not a wear-and-tear disease, so you don't need to be afraid of using the joints that have pain. In fact, they have found that osteoarthritis is caused by slow, low-grade inflammation in the body that slowly destroys the cartilage.

What causes this inflammation? Certainly, there are genetic factors, but other factors also include the presence of adipokines, which are pro-inflammatory substances produced by adipose tissue, known as fat tissue. Osteoarthritis is also more frequent in joints that have had a trauma or another inflammatory arthritis, such as rheumatoid arthritis.

To help reduce this low-grade inflammation, you can:

1. Reduce fat tissue in your body.

2. Start an anti-inflammatory diet.

3. Move your body to increase the lubrication of the joints.

The types of exercises that I recommend for people with osteoarthritis are lubrication, aerobics, weight-bearing and stretching. These are explained below.

LAWS EXERCISES FOR OSTEOARTHRITIS

L	Lubrication
A	Aerobics
W	Weight-bearing
S	Stretching and strengthening

WHY LAWS EXERCISES ARE IMPORTANT

First, you must understand why the LAWS exercises are important. When people understand why they are doing an exercise, they do it and feel motivated to keep doing it regularly.

LUBRICATION is necessary because the joint produces a liquid called synovial fluid. The fluid is produced when we move the joint and put weight on it. The synovial fluid is responsible for the nutrition of the cartilage. The cartilage is a thin layer that covers the bones to form a slippery surface, so the bones will absorb the shock and move smoothly by reducing friction. Lubrication is essential, especially in the morning. Many of my patients have morning stiffness. At night, they don't move their joints, and then there is not much synovial fluid production and the fluid tends to get thicker. This is what causes stiff and creaky joints.

WATCH MY VIDEO ON LAWS EXERCISES FOR HIP AND KNEE OSTEOPOROSIS

I recommend you do the lubrication exercises in the morning, before you get out of bed. This will help to warm up the joints, improve range of motion and break down any thickness of the synovial fluid.

You can do the other exercises, aerobics, weight-bearing and stretching exercises during the day.

AEROBICS EXERCISES are important to maintain a good cardiovascular system. Aerobic exercises are any type of exercise that increases the heart rate and respiratory rate. This may include walking briskly, dancing, biking and swimming. Talk to your doctor to make sure you don't have any restrictions on doing aerobic activity.

WEIGHT-BEARING EXERCISES are crucial for people with osteoarthritis and osteoporosis. The main advantages of weight-bearing exercises are that they reduce pain in the joint and help maintain the calcium in the bones, especially important for people who also have osteoporosis.

WATCH MY VIDEO ON LAWS EXERCISES FOR ANKLE OSTEOPOROSIS

STRETCHING is vital to maintain flexibility and a good range of motion in the joints that have osteoarthritis. When people have joint pain, they tend to protect the joint and use it less and less. Then the muscles get shortened and stiff. The tendons, ligaments and joint capsules all get very tight. It is essential to gently stretch the structures around the joints.

Exercises for myofascial pain syndrome

Myofascial pain syndrome (MPS) is pain in the muscles and fascia, the membrane that covers the muscles. It is characterized by trigger points, which are small painful areas that cause radiating pain when provoked by muscle contraction, stretching or external pressure. The pain can be reproduced by activating these trigger points.

Although MPS can progress to central sensitization and lead to fibromyalgia in people with predisposing factors, it is not the same thing as fibromyalgia.

The treatment of MPS involves identifying factors that cause and prolong the pain. The trigger points can be eliminated by relaxing the muscle and increasing the blood flow.

Underlying factors usually include:

WATCH MY VIDEO ON SSAR EXERCISES FOR NECK PAIN

- Bad posture, abnormal walking, repetitive movements, joint instability
- Constriction of muscles, as caused by a purse strap, tight bra or belt; tight scars
- Nutritional deficiencies, as in a lack of vitamin D, folate or minerals
- Metabolic or hormonal inadequacies such as hypothyroidism or diabetes
- Psychological distress, including depressed mood, anxiety and tension
- Chronic infection, such as urinary tract infection
- Impaired sleep
- Nerve compression
- Environment, especially cold temperature

WATCH MY VIDEO ON SSAR EXERCISES FOR LOW BACK PAIN

WAYS TO ELIMINATE THE TRIGGER POINTS

- SSAR exercises: stretching, strengthening, aerobics (or cardio) and relaxation
- Modalities: superficial or deep heat, electrotherapy or laser
- Biofeedback, relaxation techniques, CBT for anxiety and sleep
- Manual therapies: deep massage and mobilizations
- Acupuncture, dry needling
- Injections such as local anesthetics (no botulinum toxin or steroids)
- NSAIDs and muscle relaxants, used for a short period
- Tricyclic antidepressants, used for a more extended period

WATCH MY VIDEO ON SSAR EXERCISES FOR THORACIC PAIN

- Avoiding drugs such as opioids, benzodiazepines and baclofen
- Better ergonomics, workstation, environment temperature and shoes
- Improved sleep position, sleep hygiene

SSAR EXERCISES FOR MYOFASCIAL PAIN SYNDROME

S	Stretching
S	Strengthening
A	Aerobics
R	Relaxation

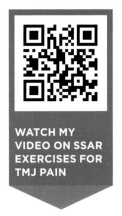

WATCH MY VIDEO ON SSAR EXERCISES FOR TMJ PAIN

Relaxation exercises

When we talk about relaxation exercises, we cannot separate relaxation of the mind from the body. The benefits of relaxation exercises include:

- Reduced muscle tension
- Reduced sympathetic nervous system activity
- Increased parasympathetic nervous system activity
- Lower blood pressure and blood sugars
- Slower heart rate and respiratory rate
- Improve digestion, sleep and concentration

> We cannot separate relaxation of the mind from the relaxation of the body.

In addition to the square breathing exercise that I described in *Step 2: Control Your Emotions*, there are many other relaxation exercises. You can find many professionals who teach these techniques, including physicians, psychotherapists, physiotherapists, complementary and alternative medicine practitioners and social workers.

Try the techniques listed on the following page and find out which one works best for you.

"Our mind has the tendency to wander away and to worry about things; that is why mindfulness is important, to bring our mind to the here and now."

RELAXATION TECHNIQUES

PROGRESSIVE MUSCLE RELAXATION	This technique involves tensing and relaxing muscle groups. It helps to notice the difference between tensed and relaxed muscles. Starting with your head and going down to your feet, tense the muscles for about 5 seconds, then relax for 30 seconds. Then go to the next muscle group — shoulders, arms, torso, abdomen, gluteus, thighs, legs and feet. You may also start from your feet and progress up.
VISUALIZATION	This technique involves imagination using the senses. Choose a quiet spot, close your eyes and visualize a calm and peaceful place. Imagine the smells, colors, shapes, sizes, sounds and textures. Focus on the present and think positive and pleasant thoughts.
BREATHING	Choose a breathing technique you are familiar with. It could be the square breathing that I explained on page 102, or something else.
AQUA THERAPY	Water-based exercises stimulate the skin through temperature and touch. This can be accomplished with a warm bath, cold shower, swimming or aqua fitness.
PRAYER	Choose a quiet place, close your eyes and practice your prayers. Focus on gratitude, cast away your fears, offer compassion to yourself and to others, think about your life's purposes and how to help others in need.
MEDITATION	Meditation is a simple technique that has been practiced for thousands of years. It is not about emptying the mind, but instead, filling the mind with focused attention. The focus can be on a particular object, thought or activity. Mind wandering is normal, especially when a person is starting to meditate. With practice, it is possible to learn and avoid mind wandering.
MINDFULNESS	There are various guided mindfulness meditations available. They instruct the individual to focus on the present without judging. It may include grounding through sensations, breathing and body movements.

Important to remember: Check with your doctor or psychologist if you have a history of post-traumatic stress disorder (PTSD) before you start mindfulness or meditation.

Exercises in the water

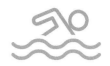

Aqua therapy, hydro gymnastics, aqua fitness, swimming, water polo and recreational swimming are excellent methods to alleviate pain from osteoarthritis, muscle spasms, myofascial pain and fibromyalgia.

Water provides many benefits to people who want to exercise for pain relief:

- It involves the whole body, all your joints and muscles, when you are immersed from the neck down.
- It provides resistance to movements, thereby increasing muscle power and strength.
- In the water, you can relax and do breathing exercises and this will activate the parasympathetic nervous system.
- Even when you are simply walking inside a pool, you are doing tremendous aerobic exercises, which are extremely important to provide oxygen to the muscles, tendons, bones and all the organs of your body.

I am not a big fan of cold water, but I have patients who swim in the waters of the Great Lakes, and they tell me that it is excellent for their various types of pains. And the Great Lakes are very cold, even in the summer.

The water temperature is not super important; what matters is if you like it or not. Some people with fibromyalgia prefer warmer water temperatures of 91 to 97°F (33 to 36°C).

I recommend you start doing exercises immersed in the water at least twice a week, for three months. It may take that long before you start seeing any benefits to your pain. Keep at it. Initially, your body will get tired, and you may have more pain. That is probably delayed-onset muscle soreness, which goes away in two days. It is the expected normal pain that we feel in our muscles when we start exercising muscles that have been resting for a long time.

"Water provides many benefits to people who want to exercise for pain relief."

Modalities

When I talk about modalities, I am referring to physical modalities, that is, therapeutic tools such as temperature, pressure, light, sound or electricity. Heat and cold are excellent temperature modalities. (I also include orthotics and ergonomics under modalities, although they are not really a physical modality.)

COLD is used to reduce acute inflammation. It constricts the blood vessels and reduces the blood flow to the affected area. This is good when there is swelling and redness in the area, as with an acute fracture, sprain or muscle tear. Cold can also stop the electrical transmission in the peripheral nerves, therefore blocking the nerves from carrying information about pain to the spinal cord. If you apply ice for more than 20 minutes to an area, that area becomes anesthetized and you can't feel pain.

HEAT is used to treat chronic pain, especially pain from the muscles. It relaxes your muscles and enables you to do stretching and strengthening exercises more effectively. Heat does not anesthetize the skin, but it does provide some relief through neurological mechanisms. It can be applied with a hot water bag, a heating pad, hot towel or topical creams.

LIGHT therapy is used for its properties of superficial heat (infrared) and laser therapy. A simple way to be exposed to infrared is by taking sun baths. Laser therapy has to be administered by a healthcare professional. Laser is sometimes is used for tendon and muscle repairs, but these are usually for acute sports injuries. For chronic pain, there are few reasons to use laser therapy, as the tissues have healed already.

> Music therapy is a great way to relax the mind and the muscles, reduce stress and improve sleep quality.

SOUND therapy has its place in the treatment of chronic pain. Some studies show that music therapy is a great way to relax the mind and the muscles, reduce stress and improve sleep quality. Another way to use sound for therapy is by administration of binaural beats. These are a type of sound illusion created in the brain when you listen to two tones with slightly different frequencies at the same time. This sound illusion can be used to train the brain to reduce some brain activity involved in pain and stress. Another use of sound is by application of therapeutic ultrasound to muscles and tendons. These sound waves will produce deep heat and help heal injuries. Again, this is helpful in acute injuries and not so much for chronic pain.

ELECTRICITY can be used to modify neuronal activity. There are a variety of electrical nerve and muscle stimulations. One of them is transcutaneous electrical nerve stimulation, or TENS. Modern TENS machines are the same size as a cell phone and can be carried around and turned on frequently and for hours at a time during the day. TENS is an electrical current that competes with painful impulses. If there is nociceptive pain in a body part, there will be electrical impulses from that part to the spinal cord. If you apply TENS to the nerve that is carrying that information from the periphery to the spinal cord, then the TENS current blocks the pain and your brain only receives the information about the TENS current, which is a little buzz, but not uncomfortable. Unfortunately, TENS does not work well for neuropathic or nociplastic pain.

TAPING is the application of sticky tape to the skin right above the area that is painful. Many athletes use this technique to help them heal from acute sports-related injuries. If there is already nociplastic pain, then taping will not be enough to provide any practical benefit.

SPLINTS, BRACES, ORTHOTICS, ERGONOMIC CHAIRS, ERGONOMIC DESKS, PILLOWS AND MATTRESSES: These are all objects that can be used to provide proper positioning of the body. They help to avoid aggravation of pain by improving posture, alignment, reducing muscle tension or pressure on some body parts. I recommend you get a proper pillow and mattress appropriate for your body composition. These do not need to be expensive!

DO NOT WASTE YOUR MONEY ON ANY OF THIS EQUIPMENT!

- Whole body vibration machine
- Electrical massage gadgets
- Collars to immobilize the neck
- Lumbar corsets
- Home-based traction for lumbar or cervical spine
- Water mattresses for back pain

Manual Therapy

Manual therapies involve some sort of hands-on therapy, or the application of pressure to the body using a machine or device. The three major types of manual therapies are massage, mobilization and manipulation.

There are many different techniques practiced by physiotherapists, occupational therapists, chiropractors, osteopaths and massage therapists. They often integrate manual therapies with other methods that involve heat, cold, electrical or light therapy.

There is evidence that manual therapies work for some kinds of chronic pain, including neck and lower back pain, myofascial pain and arthritis-related pain. Unfortunately, there is no evidence that manual therapies are helpful for neuropathic or nociplastic pain.

Manual therapies are passive modalities and should never replace active interventions such as movement-based or mind-body exercises. Also, manual therapy can be quite costly. I usually suggest my patients use a session of manual therapy when they have a flare-up or after they have tried other active modalities and they still have pain. I don't recommend they keep going to manual therapists to prevent flares or for maintenance when their pain can be managed with home-based modalities such as a heating pad.

DO IT YOURSELF

I teach many of my patients to do self-massage. You can learn how to find your trigger points, how to get rid of muscle knots and how to use some inexpensive equipment to provide local pressure on your body. I recommend a hard foam roller for shoulder, back, hip, thigh and leg pains. You can also try a J-shape cane or roll on an old tennis ball to apply pressure to hard-to-reach spots on your back.

Medications

We explored medications in the previous chapter. All medicines have adverse effects and they should be used only after the other four of the 5Ms have not provided enough pain relief, and only as advised by your doctor or pharmacist.

CONCLUSION

How many tools do you have in your toolbox? You can make a list and carry it with you. The next time your pain flares up, remember to open your toolbox and start with the safest tools.

KEY POINTS TO REMEMBER

- There are many ways to reduce the intensity of pain. Learn what works for you.
- Prepare yourself for a flare-up and use it as an opportunity to try new strategies to reduce pain.
- Remember the 5Ms and try to have as many tools in each M as possible.
- Don't get discouraged if a tool that worked yesterday is not working today. Stay optimistic.
- The best interventions for chronic pain are the ones that you can do to yourself. This is self-management. Prioritize active interventions instead of passive treatments.
- Try to combine interventions for the mind and body.
- Remember that humans are beings with a bio-psycho-social-spiritual nature. All of these elements are interconnected and can affect each other.
- Movement is more than just exercise. You can move anywhere. Motion is lotion to your joints.
- If you don't know where the start with movement, think FITT for frequency, intensity, time and type.
- Pick the exercises that are best for your condition. Don't forget that relaxation exercises are good for everyone.
- Osteoarthritis and osteoporosis are common among older adults, and both get better with movement.
- Modalities and manual therapies can be quite expensive, but in most cases, you can find low-cost solutions.

LOOKING AHEAD

Move on to *Step 8: Focus on Your Goals*, because the world needs you to reach the top of the mountain. You will see how you can conquer pain step by step by setting SMARTer goals.

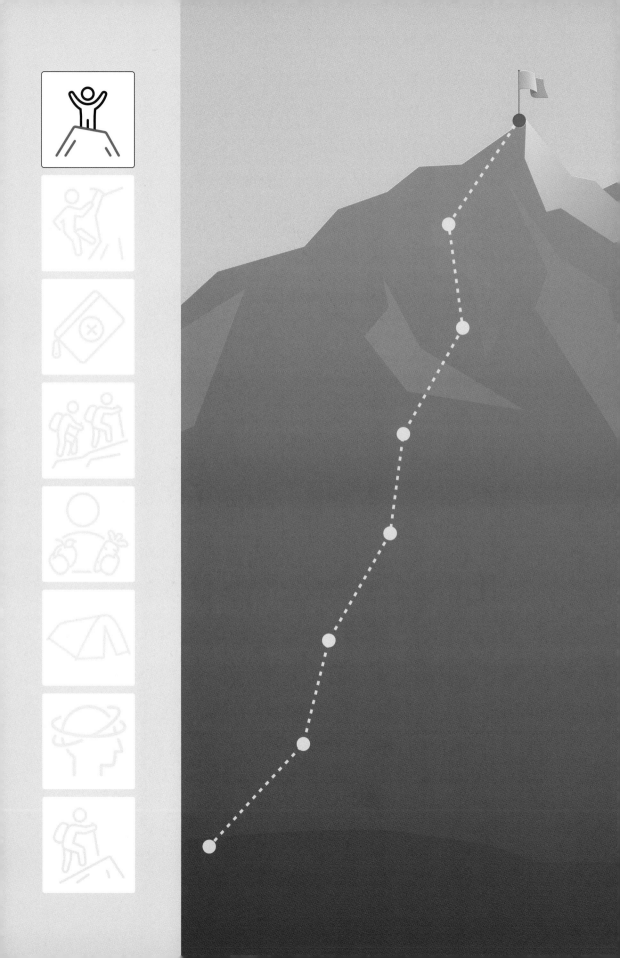

Focus on Your Goals

The primary goal of every mountaineer is to reach the top. If they don't have a clear focus, they will end up wandering aimlessly and never reach the top. They may also have other smaller goals throughout their journey. For example, they may want to improve their physical fitness, see places that nobody sees and take amazing photographs.

In this chapter, we will imagine what the future looks like when you have reached the top of the mountain. I will show you the **pain trajectory**, or the course that pain may take in the lifetime of a person. We will review some of the ways in which you can change your pain trajectory. This book is full of strategies that can lead to a favorable pain trajectory! We'll discuss how important it is to have secondary goals. We'll see how setting SMARTer goals can help you to prioritize what you really want and keep you moving forward. And we will look at ways to manage pain flare-ups and keep them from throwing you off-course.

The Pain Trajectory

The figure below shows one person's quality of life over time. In this case, their quality of life is declining as a result of chronic pain. When their pain started, this person had a good quality of life, but over time, the quality of life was decreasing, and today they would say their quality of life is lower than when the pain started.

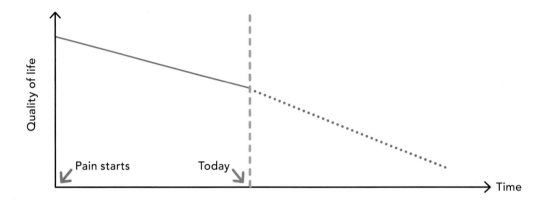

When a person with chronic pain looks at their past, they see the years of having pain most of the time, even when they did everything their doctors and therapists told them to do. Even when they did all that, and invested time and money in finding relief, still they see their pain interfering with their quality of life and their lives drifting away.

So, what do they do? They project their future. If the past was all going downhill, then they think that their future will continue that downhill course. And then they get desperate, because they can't imagine how they will be able to endure a situation worse than their pain today.

> Chase your dreams, not a cure for your pain.

Their future projection is based on their past experiences. They don't believe they can change the trajectory of their pain. They cannot see any solution or imagine how they will get out of the dark hole of pain. They project a future of suffering, depression and loss.

When a person realizes that their future is in their hands, and that they can change their pain trajectory, they feel hopeful for the future. This hope is the spark needed to change the future.

What if it doesn't work?

"What if it doesn't work?" is a question I have heard before. Many patients are terrified of trying something different, believing that they will get better and then being disappointed. They are weary of disappointments. They are tired of failed attempts. Many give up trying again.

I have seen young patients in their twenties and thirties who are in this situation. They don't want to spend more energy in trying another new approach. They want passive treatments, such as a pill, a massage, injections, or even surgery or brain stimulators.

The brain is the most powerful organ in our body. It controls everything else. What you put in your mind controls the rest of your body. That is why it is important to focus on your goals. If your brain is occupied with your goals, it will have little space to focus on pain and suffering.

If you change the way you see pain, the way you see your future and the way you approach treatments, it is possible to conquer pain and change your future. You may need a different kind of healthcare team. Instead of medications, injections and surgeries, you need a life coach, a counselor, a wellness approach, a functional medicine specialist, an integrative pain team. All of these changes and people will help you to do what have I explained throughout this book.

> If you change the way you see pain, the way you see your future and the way you approach treatments, it is possible to conquer pain and change your future.

POSSIBLE WAYS TO CHANGE YOUR PAIN TRAJECTORY

MAYBE ...	TAKE THE NEXT STEP
... your pain is mostly coming from a nociplastic origin. It is primary chronic pain and not secondary to something that is broken in your body. It is quite possible that the nociceptive or neuropathic pains have healed and they are not contributing to the pain you are feeling now. A knowledgeable doctor will be able to tell you what kind of pain you have.	See *What Is Pain?* pages 20–39; *Getting a Diagnosis*, pages 40–59; and *Step 1: Retrain Your Brain*, pages 60–77.
... you are malnourished and need to improve your nutritional status.	See *Step 4: Fix Your Diet*, pages 134–157.
... you need to change your sleep habits and improve your sleep efficiency.	See *Step 3: Get Quality Sleep*, pages 120–133.

MAYBE ...	TAKE THE NEXT STEP
... you need to stop being afraid of pain.	See *Step 2: Control Your Emotions*, pages 78–119.
... you need to get moving again. Even if it hurts, you need to move your body.	See *Step 2: Control Your Emotions*, pages 78–119; and *Step 7: Make Room in Your Toolbox*, pages 216–239.
... you need to stop blaming other people for your pain and suffering. Forgive, forget and move on with your life.	See *Step 2: Control Your Emotions*, pages 78–119.
... you need to taper and stop all your pain medications. Please check with your doctor and pharmacist if there are any pain medications that you could discontinue or decrease the dosage.	See *Step 5: Get Help from Others*, pages 158–183; and *Step 6: Check Your Medicine Cabinet*, pages 184–215.
... you need to stop chasing a diagnosis, stop asking for X-rays, CT scans, MRIs, blood tests and expensive exams.	See *Getting a Diagnosis*, pages 40–59.
... you need to stop passive treatment modalities such as massages, TENS, manipulations, injections and surgeries and start a self-management program in which you are the one treating your own body and mind.	See *Step 7: Make Room in Your Toolbox*, pages 216–239.
... you need to offer help instead of asking help. Start volunteering, find a person who needs help and offer to do something for them.	See *Step 5: Get Help from Others*, pages 158–183; and *Step 7: Make Room in Your Toolbox*, pages 216–239.
... it would help if you saw yourself differently. You have had pain for so long that you identify most with other people who have pain. When you introduce yourself, you say, "I'm a person with chronic pain." Pain does not need to define you. You are more than your pain.	See *Step 1: Retrain Your Brain*, pages 60–77.
... you need to stop being around other people who are struggling with pain, and start being around people who have conquered pain. Find someone who has conquered pain and ask them what they did and how they changed their trajectory.	See *Step 5: Get Help from Others*, pages 158–183.

Don't go too fast

You might be excited to start changing things in your life right now. Don't try to make too many changes simultaneously or go too fast. Allow time for your body, mind and soul to adjust.

MAKE A LIST OF YOUR PRIORITIES RIGHT NOW

Where do you want to start? Break your plan into small, bite-size goals. You can always adjust your plan. You can slow or accelerate as you go. (We discuss SMARTer goals later in this chapter.)

It is easier to keep climbing than it is to start climbing when you are stopped. The important thing is that you are doing something, you are moving toward the peak of the mountain. The speed you travel at is not the critical element; it is more important to not get stuck.

> When you live your dreams, your pain will lose importance and become so insignificant that you will barely notice it.

PACE YOURSELF

Pacing means that you are doing your activities at your limits. You don't need to compare yourself with another person who has chronic pain. They may be going faster or slower than you. You need to compare you with yourself yesterday. Did you move an inch from yesterday? Good! Did you move a yard from yesterday? Good. It doesn't matter how much you moved, as long as you are not giving up and stopping.

FIND THE RIGHT BALANCE BETWEEN TOO MUCH AND TOO LITTLE ACTIVITY

Too much will put more stress on your body and mind. Too little will not get you to your goal. Don't overdo one day and then do nothing the next day. This see-saw pattern is not helpful. Schedule some resting time during your day. And don't rest too much. As we saw in *Step 3: Get Quality Sleep*, longer naps in the afternoon reduce the quality of sleep at night. But a short nap of less than 30 minutes in the afternoon can be very refreshing. Also remember that some caffeine in the morning is helpful to wake up the brain, but too much caffeine during the day and in the evening will disrupt sleep at night and may cause other serious health side effects.

Here are some suggestions for resting and distracting activities that you can schedule during your day. Set a time to begin and finish these activities.

- Listen to music, radio or an audiobook.
- Talk to someone. Visit a friend, a neighbor, a community center, a religious place or a seniors' residence.
- Watch a TV show, a movie or a sports game.
- Read a book, the newspaper or some posts on social media.
- Do a craft, such as drawing, painting, crocheting or knitting.
- Write in your journal, or write a letter or email to a friend or a post on social media.
- Play with a pet, or play a board game, a video game or a game on a tablet or cellphone.
- Organize a drawer, wardrobe, kitchen, a box; recycle stuff and donate.
- Shop online, go to a local store or go to a large mall.
- Visit a garden center, flower shop, botanic garden, local library, museum or park.

How Will You Know If You Have Reached the Top of the Mountain?

If the mountain climber has to call the rescue helicopter because they can't get to the top of the mountain, they should not let this stop their career as an alpinist. They still achieved a lot of other goals on their way up. They learned a lot and they will be able to use their knowledge to try again. The important thing is to keep trying. They may fail one, two or three mountains, but if they keep trying, one day they will reach the top of another mountain.

The goal of every patient that I have with chronic pain is to eliminate their pain. They want to go back to a life without pain. I tell them there is a possibility that will happen. In my 30 years of experience as a pain doctor, I've seen that, not rarely, but many times.

Yet most people do not go back to what they were before; they rediscover and redesign their new identity. They acknowledge that pain has modified them, but they are now more resilient and stronger.

You know when you have reached the top of the mountain when you have all the tools you need to live a fulfilling life and you stop searching for another treatment that will have the answer to your problems.

What are your goals?

Let's do an exercise. On your journey to the top of the mountain, if we cannot eliminate pain, what are other things you want to achieve in life that you can count as successes?

1 Can you list ten secondary goals?

2 Go back to the beginning of your journal, where I asked you how would you know if you conquered pain. What did you write?

3 Do you still agree with what you wrote? Or would you change your goal?

It is okay to change and refine your goals.

I will give you a hand. I'll show you how you can write meaningful, attainable goals, large and small. No goal is too small. You are in control of your own goals.

Have you arrived at the top? Can you celebrate now — or not yet? If you don't have goals, you will never know if you have conquered your mountain.

How SMART Are Your Goals?

Have you heard of SMART goals? Well, you need SMARTer goals. These are goals that are specific, measurable, attainable, relevant, time-bound, evaluable and revisable.

> No goal is too small.

If you don't know how to start, you may need to get help from a professional. Occupational therapists, physical therapists, social workers, psychologists are all trained in how to help people to set their SMARTer goals. I've provided some examples here to give you an idea of what can be done, but there are infinite possibilities.

SMARTER GOALS

S	Specific
M	Measurable
A	Attainable
R	Relevant
T	Time-bound
E	Evaluable
R	Revisable

Three examples of SMARTer goals

KATE'S SMARTER GOALS

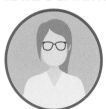 Kate is a 25-year-old woman with chronic neck pain of myofascial origin (caused by tight muscle fibers). She works as a receptionist in a small office and her goal is to study to become a bilingual medical secretary. She wants to get a better paid job so she can work part-time and be able to raise a family. She needs to work during the day and study on evenings and weekends. Working at a computer station and studying with books has made her neck pain much worse. She is worried she will not be able to fulfill her dream of advancing her career and getting a better paid job.

This was her not-so-smart goal: "One day, I will get a job as a bilingual medical secretary."

Here are Kate's revised SMARTer goals: "By the end of this month I will finish studying chapter 1 of the textbook required to get my certification as a bilingual medical secretary. If I study one chapter per month, it will take me 36 months to finish studying and be able to write the exams. I will take breaks during my working day to do the stretching, strengthening and relaxation exercises. I will walk 30 minutes every day to complete my aerobics exercises minimum requirement. I will sleep eight hours every night and I will eat healthy this month."

Let's analyze Kate's SMARTer goals:

S	Her goal is specific because she knows what she has to do. She has to read one chapter of the book. She knows which book it is. She already has the book.
M	Her goal is measurable because it is only one chapter per month.
A	She set her goals very low. She probably could achieve this goal in one week.
R	Her goal is relevant, as it will allow her to write the exams to get the job she wants.

T	One month is enough time for her to study the chapter really well.
E	She can evaluate if this is the right goal for her or not. Maybe studying by herself is not the best way to study for the exams. Perhaps she will need to register at a school or an online course or join a study group.
R	If necessary, she can make readjustments to her goal. If she finishes the chapters in one week instead of one month, she can revise her plan. Or, if she needs more time to study one chapter, she can also give herself more time.

JOHN'S SMARTER GOALS

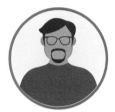 John is a 52-year-old man with chronic low back pain. He is a truck driver, happily married and a father of four children ranging from 10 to 20 years of age. He uses multiple medications to manage his constant daily pain: duloxetine, acetaminophen, ibuprofen, pregabalin and oxycodone. He is worried about his ability to drive and keep his job. His boss has seen him taking naps during the breaks and has threatened to fire him because he seems too sedated. His coworkers are spreading rumors he is addicted and dangerous to be around. He has had some angry outbursts at work. He says he is not himself and he doesn't see any other way to alleviate his pain. His not-so-smart goals are: "I want to keep my job to provide for my family, and I want my boss to respect me and my coworkers to stop bullying me."

Here are John's revised SMARTer goals: "I take so many medications and I am still in pain. I will make an appointment with my doctor next week and tell him/her that I need to reduce my pain medications. I will tell my doctor that I want to start reducing the oxycodone first, then we will try the other medications. I know this will make me more alert and less groggy. I will talk to my boss and tell him that I am making changes to my pain medications so I can be more alert. I will play soccer with my kids twice a week to add some physical exercise to my life. My kids always ask me to play with them and I always find an excuse and blame the pain for not playing with them. I will make these changes for one month and then, if I can achieve these goals, I'll keep them and add a few more. My next goal will probably be to try to quit smoking."

Let's analyze John's SMARTer goals:

S	He will book an appointment with his doctor and ask the doctor to start tapering oxycodone. This is a very strategic goal toward his bigger goal of continuing to drive a truck without causing any serious injury to himself or anyone else.
M	He will see the doctor next week and they will start an opioid tapering plan. The time that will take to taper his oxycodone will depend on various factors. It may take weeks, months or years, but the important is that these goals can be measured.
A	It is possible to reduce pain medications, especially if he is motivated and willing to try other modalities to treat his low back pain. Playing soccer with his kids will help both physical and mental health components.
R	These goals are relevant for him to keep his job and regain the trust of his boss. He has demonstrated responsibility for his actions and that he is concerned about the safety of his coworkers too.
T	These goals can be achieved in the time frame he established.
E	He can evaluate if these goals are appropriate or not. His doctor may suggest that they taper another drug first.
R	He can readjust his goals. For example, instead of playing with his children twice a week, he can increase it to three times a week, or reduce to once a week.

CAROL'S SMARTER GOALS

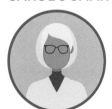

Carol is a 79-year-old widow, a retired teacher. She lives alone in a two-story house and doesn't get out of the house much. She loves traveling, reading and visiting museums. She has osteoarthritis that affects her hands, shoulders, hips, knees and feet. She has fibromyalgia and migraines. She doesn't take any pain medications because she has adverse side effects with all of them. She is very sensitive to noise, bright light and chemicals.

Her not-so-smart goals are: "I want to travel to all the cities in Europe and buy books to bring home and read them."

Here are Carol's SMARTer goals: "I will go to the local library once a week and borrow one book to read. I will read one book per week. I will ask one of my children, grandchildren or a friend to take me to a local museum once a month. I will try to walk at the museum for one hour and then, if I can't do that, I will ask them for a wheeled chair to finish seeing the museum. My city only has one museum, so, for next month I will arrange a trip to another city to visit a museum there. I will try to do a different city every month. I will bring my sunglasses in case the light is too bright, and I will bring my ear mufflers in case the noise is too bothersome. I will do 30 minutes of stair exercises at home to increase my exercise tolerance. I think if I keep doing this, in two years I will be able to book a one-week trip to Portugal or Spain (but not both)."

Let's analyze Carol's SMARTer goals:

S	She is starting with small goals to get to her bigger goal. Going to the local library once a week is a very specific task. Going to the museum once a month is very specific too.
M	She can track her progress toward once a week going to the library and once a month going to the museum. She can also track the 30 minutes of daily stairs exercises.
A	Her goals can be achieved and they are under her control.
R	These goals are relevant to give her the confidence that she needs before she goes on the trip to Europe.
T	These goals have a reasonable time frame. She can keep a calendar to track these activities.
E	She can evaluate if these goals are working or not. She could modify them if she thinks they will not help her to go on a trip to Europe.
R	She can readjust the frequency of trips to the library and to a museum, and the amount of time and frequency of stair exercises.

Set your own SMARTer goals

Let's do an exercise.

1. Get your journal and write down your own SMARTer goals.

2. Remember to make them **S**pecific, **M**easurable, **A**ttainable, **R**elevant, **T**ime-bound, **E**valuable and **R**evisable.

I am a big fan of Rick Hansen, from British Columbia. He became paraplegic at a young age and he does so much for people with disabilities.

"Lean on medical professionals, family and friends as you strive to achieve as much recovery as possible, and have hope for the advancement of treatment care and cures. Live each day to its fullest. Try to see that there is love, beauty and meaning in spite of pain, suffering and challenges. Realize that a full and productive life is possible if barriers are removed. Look for examples of progress and role models of what is possible to help inspire you to see your full potential. Recognize that you are not alone. As you adjust to your new reality, it may be hard to believe in the beginning that you will be providing inspiration to those who you come into contact with. By moving forward to reclaim your life, and make the best of it, you will be making a difference."

— Rick Hansen, www.rickhansen.com

When you achieve your goals, don't forget to celebrate!
Take a picture of you achieving your SMARTer
goal and tag me on social media with this hashtag:
#ConquerPainWithDrFurlan.

"The way we react to a situation can be more dangerous to our body than the situation itself."

How to Manage a Flare-up

Flare-ups will happen. You need to be prepared for these episodes or worsening pain. They can happen anytime without warning. You may be doing everything right, taking good care of your body, your emotions and your relationships, and then it happens. You have a bad day, a bad week or even a bad month! It throws you off. It distracts you and kills your enthusiasm for taking care of yourself.

1. Check with your doctor

The first thing to do is to check with your clinician to make sure there are no complications such as nerve compression, infection, fracture, tumor (cancer) or acute inflammation. We call these NIFTI.

If there are no symptoms or physical examination signs of NIFTI, you can be reassured that this pain is not a cause for worry. It will not harm your body and it will not get worse. It is a signal that is being felt at the brain. And, as you have already learned, this signal can be amplified by your thoughts, emotions and fears.

NIFTI

N	Nerve compression
I	Infection
F	Fracture
T	Tumor
I	Inflammation

2. Try to identify a precipitating factor

What happened when this pain flared up? Use the following checklist:

☑ **Body movement:** Did you carry excess weight? Did you turn quickly? Did you do more exercises than you usually do?

☑ **Lack of body movement:** Did you stop doing your regular physical activity? Did you stop doing the exercises that have helped you to conquer your pain?

☑ *Emotional stress:* Was there any situation at home or at work? Did you watch news that was disturbing to you? Did you get angry or frustrated? Are you afraid of something? Are you worried about a current situation or about the future?

☑ *Other factors outside of your control:* These could be weather changes or the flu.

3. Use all the tools in your toolbox

1. Use the non-medication tools first. If you condition your brain to use medications for flares, it will be hard to disconnect those neurons later and undo those synapses.

2. Give yourself time to wait for the flare to stop.

3. Inform only those people who need to know about your flare. This could be your spouse, your caregiver or your boss. Avoid telling people who do not know how to help you, or those who will be worried about you and will not know what to do. They can be a source of more anxiety to you.

4. Keep a positive attitude. Remember the previous flare episodes and how you did well to overcome them. They didn't last forever. They went away. This current episode will go away too.

5. Try to keep moving as much as possible. Avoid prolonged periods of bed rest or inactivity.

6. Avoid filling your mind with bad news and pessimistic thoughts.

7. Try staying creative. This could involve singing, playing a musical instrument, dancing, painting, crocheting, knitting, organizing your house, writing letters and any other crafts that you may enjoy.

8. Don't listen to anyone who brings negative messages to you, especially if they say you are failing to take care of yourself, that your journey to wellness is not working or that you will end up crippled.

CONCLUSION

If you change the way you see pain, the way you see your future and the way you approach treatments, it is possible to conquer pain and change your future. Chase your dreams, not a cure for your pain. When you live your dreams, your pain can become so insignificant that you will barely notice it.

KEY POINTS TO REMEMBER

- You can change your pain trajectory. It's not all downhill from here!
- Setting SMARTer goals can help you to prioritize what you really want and keep you moving forward. It's important to have secondary goals.
- You can plan for and manage flare-ups.

LOOKING AHEAD

You are almost done. In the next chapter, you will see that you are prepared to face chronic pain head-on and conquer it.

Conclusion

You have reached the end of this book. Well done!

I recommend you keep this book and your journal handy to remind you of your goals, the tools that you have and how you can conquer your chronic pain. You may also watch the videos on my YouTube channel for more tips and information.

Your past doesn't need to predict your future

Today is the day to start making significant changes to your life, not just your pain. Your quality of life can improve. You may never be the same person you were before you were affected by chronic pain. But you can become a better person, more resilient and self-sufficient. Your pain trajectory does not have to be all downhill.

Today we have modern techniques to treat nociceptive and neuropathic pain very effectively. And there are ways to manage and overcome nociplastic pain.

Don't let nociplastic pain linger in your life too long. Acknowledge the nature and origin of your pain. If it is nociplastic pain, then embrace it, learn how to retrain your pain system and make options for a healthier lifestyle that includes more self-management approaches.

I find that people who lose the fear of the pain can handle the mountains much better. They keep their life as normal as possible. It seems that the pain does not have nearly as strong an influence on them anymore.

When you are ready and willing to make changes, you can alter the course of your pain trajectory so that it looks more like the figure below.

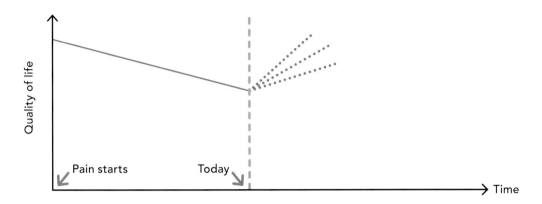

The mountaineer is back at home! Mission accomplished. They are looking at their photos and their notes, sharing stories about their adventure with family and friends. And planning for the next journey.

Did the mountain disappear? No, the mountain is still there. It may not be a challenge to this mountaineer, but it will be a challenge to another one. And the climber from our story will undoubtedly face a different mountain, but now with more experience and expertise. Our mountaineer is thinking of coaching other novice mountaineers how to climb their mountains.

Every person has a different mountain and a different story to tell. Here are some stories from fellow conquerors:

- Pamela, 46-year-old female: "I have chronic migraine. I was able to conquer migraine by improving my sleep and changing my diet. I still have days with migraines, but they are less frequent and less intense. And when I do have a migraine, I know which tools from my toolbox work best for me."
- Lucia, 62-year-old female: "I have recently been diagnosed with fibromyalgia. I was scared. I conquered my fear of being disabled and useless by working with my emotions, getting knowledge from reliable sources, being prepared when I visit my family doctor and by contributing to an online group of patients with fibromyalgia."

- Hamad, 59-year-old male: "I have had neuropathic pain even since I had a stroke. I conquered this pain by adhering to the course of medications that the doctor prescribed to me. Before, I was not using them properly. I also recognize that when I am tired, angry and frustrated, my pain is worse. I feel a lot of relief when I practice meditation."

You will have ups and downs. There might be relapses in your pain. The pain may come back the same, worse or better than before. We don't know when the next mountain will show up in your life.

But now, you are more equipped to conquer the next mountain. Usually, what happens is that you will not be so afraid of the pain next time, because now you know what to do and what to think.

WATCH A TESTIMONIAL VIDEO

CASE STUDY

SYLVIO AND THE LOCAL COMMUNITY CENTER

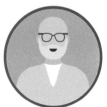

Sylvio is an 84-year-old retired construction worker. He has rheumatoid arthritis, chronic low back pain and neuropathic pain in his feet. He was on many painkillers that did not eliminate his pain. They also made him feel tired, dizzy and constipated.

We helped him to taper the opioids slowly and he stopped using them completely. He said his pain was still the same, but he felt more alert and not dizzy or constipated anymore.

Sylvio acknowledged that he would have this pain for the rest of his life, so he started participating in aqua therapy with a group of friends at the local community center. He goes three or four times a week. They exercise together and then they go out to local restaurants, museums and parks. He said his quality of life is excellent and pain does not limit what he wants to do.

Engaging in regular physical activity is an excellent strategy to conquer pain, but social interactions, meaningful activities and pleasure are also extremely important tools to reward the brain for doing the right thing.

You Can Live Well with Chronic Pain, Now and in the Future

Even when you reach a point where you believe you have conquered your pain, that does not mean that your pain has gone away forever.

Is more pain inevitable? Should you be downhearted? Not at all. You are now much better equipped to conquer any future challenges.

- ☑ You have all the tools you need in your toolbox to manage a relapse or flare-up.

- ☑ You are not lost. You have a map of where to go.

- ☑ You won't feel lonely on this journey. You have people you can trust.

- ☑ You are competent, knowledgeable and an expert on your condition.

- ☑ You can mentor other people who are starting their journey with pain.

- ☑ You are prepared to conquer higher and more challenging mountains. If you face a worsening of your pain, another injury, a setback or a relapse, you can go back to your notes and tackle the problem head-on.

- ☑ You have developed endurance and resilience.

- ☑ You are not afraid of pain.

- ☑ You will not let pain dictate what you can or cannot do.

It is possible to live well with chronic pain. You are not alone. There are 100 million Americans and 7 million Canadians who live with chronic pain. You are stronger than you think.

If you have got through this book to this point, you have the energy and strength that it takes to conquer pain.

You have the power within yourself. I believe in you. Believe in yourself!

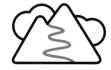

References and Resources

WHAT IS PAIN?

REFERENCES

Davis, Karen D., Herta Flor, Henry T. Greely, Gian Domenico Iannetti, Sean Mackey, Markus Ploner, Amanda Pustilnik, Irene Tracey, Rolf-Detlef Treede, and Tor D Wager. 2017. "Brain imaging tests for chronic pain: Medical, legal and ethical issues and recommendations." *Nature Reviews Neurology* 13 (10):624–638. doi:10.1038/nrneurol.2017.122

Fisher, J.P., D.T. Hassan, and N. O'Connor. 1995. *Minerva British Medical Journal* 310 (Jan):70. doi:10.1136/bmj.310.6971.70

Nijs, Jo, Paul van Wilgen, Jessica Van Oosterwijck, Miriam van Ittersum, and Mira Meeus. 2011. "How to explain central sensitization to patients with 'unexplained' chronic musculoskeletal pain: Practice guidelines." *Manual Therapy* 16 (5), 413–418. https://doi.org/10.1016/j.math.2011.04.005

Treede, Rolf-Detlef, Winfried Rief, Antonia Barke, Qasim Aziz, Michael I. Bennett, Rafael Benoliel, Milton Cohen, et al. 2015. "A classification of chronic pain for ICD-11." *Pain* 156 (6):1003–1007. doi:10.1097/j.pain.0000000000000160

WHO. 2019/2021. *International Classification of Diseases, Eleventh Revision* (ICD-11), World Health Organization (WHO)

GETTING A DIAGNOSIS

REFERENCES

Brinjikji, W., P. H. Luetmer, B. Comstock, et al. 2015. "Systematic literature review of imaging features of spinal degeneration in asymptomatic populations." *American Journal of Neuroradiology* 36 (4), 811–816. https://doi.org/10.3174/ajnr.A4173

Felitti, V. J., R. F. Anda, D. Nordenberg, et al. 1998. "Relationship of childhood abuse and household dysfunction to many of the leading causes of death in adults. The Adverse Childhood Experiences (ACE) Study." *American Journal of Preventive Medicine* 14 (4), 245–258. https://doi.org/10.1016/s0749-3797(98)00017-8

STEP 1: RETRAIN YOUR PAIN SYSTEM

REFERENCES

Ashar, Yoni K., Alan Gordon, Howard Schubiner, Christie Uipi, Karen Knight, Zachary Anderson, Judith Carlisle, et al. 2022 "Effect of Pain Reprocessing Therapy vs Placebo and Usual Care for Patients with Chronic Back Pain: A Randomized Clinical Trial." *JAMA Psychiatry* 79 (1):13–23. doi:10.1001/jamapsychiatry.2021.2669

Bagg, Matthew K., Benedict M. Wand, Aidan G. Cashin, Hopin Lee, Markus Hübscher, Tasha R. Stanton, Neil E. O'Connell, et al. 2022. "Effect of Graded Sensorimotor Retraining on Pain Intensity in Patients with Chronic Low Back Pain: A Randomized Clinical Trial. *JAMA* 328 (5):430–439. doi:10.1001/jama.2022.9930

Darnall, Beth D., Anuradha Roy, Abby L. Chen, Maisa S Ziadni, Ryan T Keane, Dokyoung S. You, Kristen Slater, et al. 2021. "Comparison of a Single-Session Pain Management Skills Intervention with a Single-Session Health Education Intervention and 8 Sessions of Cognitive Behavioral Therapy in Adults with Chronic Low Back Pain: A Randomized Clinical Trial." *JAMA Network Open* 4 (8):e2113401. doi:10.1001/jamanetworkopen.2021.13401

Kerns, Robert D., Roberta Rosenberg, Robert N. Jamison, Margaret A. Caudill, Jennifer Haythornthwaite. 1997. "Readiness to adopt a self-management approach to chronic pain: The Pain Stages of Change Questionnaire (PSOCQ)." *Pain* 72 (1–2):227–234. https://doi.org/10.1016/s0304-3959(97)00038-9

Moseley, G. Lorimer. 2005. "Is successful rehabilitation of complex regional pain syndrome due to sustained attention to the affected limb? A randomised clinical trial." *Pain* 114 (1–2):54–61. doi:10.1016/j.pain.2004.11.024

Prochaska, J. O., and C. C. DiClemente (1983). "Stages and processes of self-change of smoking: Toward an integrative model of change." *Journal of Consulting and Clinical Psychology* 51 (3), 390–395. https://doi.org/10.1037//0022-006x.51.3.390

Shapiro, Francine. 2013. *Take Control of Your Life with Self-Help Techniques from EMDR Therapy.* New York: Rodale Books

Villemure, Chantal, Marta Čeko, Valerie A. Cotton, and M. Catherine Bushnell. 2015. "Neuroprotective effects of yoga practice: age-, experience-, and frequency-dependent plasticity." *Frontiers in Human Neuroscience* 9: 281. doi:10.3389/fnhum.2015.00281

RESOURCES

Darnall, Beth. 2014. *Less Pain, Fewer Pills: Avoid the Dangers of Prescription Opioids and Gain Control over Chronic Pain.* Bull Publishing Company.

Gordon, Alan, with Alon Ziv. 2021. *The Way Out: A Revolutionary, Scientifically Proven Approach to Healing Chronic Pain.* Avery, Penguin Random House

Moseley, G. Lorimer, and David S. Butler. 2015. *The Explain Pain Handbook Protectometer.* Noigroup Publications

Schubiner, Howard, with Michael Betzold. 2010. *Unlearn Your Pain: A 28-Day Process to Reprogram Your Brain.* Pleasant Ridge, MI: Mind Body Publishing

STEP 2: CONTROL YOUR EMOTIONS

REFERENCES

American Psychiatric Association (APA). 2022. "What Is Depression?" Psychiatry.org. https://psychiatry.org/patients-families/depression/what-is-depression

Canadian Centre on Substance Use and Addiction (CCSA). 2018. "Canada's Low-Risk Alcohol Drinking Guidelines" [brochure]. Ottawa: CCSA. https://www.ccsa.ca/sites/default/files/2020-07/2012-Canada-Low-Risk-Alcohol-Drinking-Guidelines-Brochure-en_0.pdf

Spitzer, Robert L., Kurt Kroenke, Janet B. Williams, and Bernd Löwe B. 2006. "A brief measure for assessing generalized anxiety disorder: The GAD-7." *Archives of Internal Medicine* 166 (10), 1092–1097. https://doi.org/10.1001/archinte.166.10.1092

Sullivan, Michael J. L., Scott R. Bishop, and Jayne Pivik. 1995. "The Pain Catastrophizing Scale: Development and Validation." *Psychological Assessment* 7 (4): 524–532. doi:10.1037/1040-3590.7.4.524

Sullivan, Michael J. L., Heather Adams, Sharon Horan, Denise Maher, Dan Boland, and Richard Gross. 2008. "The role of perceived injustice in the experience of chronic pain and disability: scale development and validation." *Journal of Occupational Rehabilitation* 18 (3):249–61. doi:10.1007/s10926-008-9140-5

Waddell, Gordon, Mary Newton, Iain Henderson, Douglas Somerville, and Chris J. Main. 1993. "A Fear-Avoidance Beliefs Questionnaire (FABQ) and the role of fear-avoidance beliefs in chronic low back pain and disability." *Pain* 52 (2), 157–168. https://doi.org/10.1016/0304-3959(93)90127-B

Whymper, Edward. 1871. *Scrambles Among the Alps.* In Bellingham Mountaineers (2019), *Bellingham Mountaineers Basic Mountaineering Course Manual.* Page 6.

RESOURCES

Ontario Region of Narcotics Anonymous: https://www.orscna.org/

Sarno, John E. 1999. *The Mindbody Prescription: Healing the Body, Healing the Pain.* Grand Central Publishing

STEP 3: GET QUALITY SLEEP

REFERENCES

Cai, H, N. Su , W. Li, et al. 2021. "Relationship between afternoon napping and cognitive function in the ageing Chinese population." *General Psychiatry* 34:e100361. doi: 10.1136/gpsych-2020-100361

Canadian Network for Mood and Anxiety Treatment (CANMAT). 2016. *Clinical Guidelines for the Management of Adults with Major Depressive Disorder.* https://www.canmat.org/sdm_downloads/2016-depression-guidelines/

Fetveit, A., and B. Bjorvatn. 2004. "The effects of bright-light therapy on actigraphical measured sleep last for several weeks post-treatment. A study in a nursing home population." *Journal of Sleep Research* 13 (2): 153–158. https://doi.org/10.1111/j.1365-2869.2004.00396.x

Gkolias, V., A. Amaniti, A. Triantafyllou, P. Papakonstantinou, P. Kartsidis, E. Paraskevopoulos, P. D. Bamidis, L. Hadjileontiadis, and D. Kouvelas. 2020. "Reduced pain and analgesic use after acoustic binaural beats therapy in chronic pain: A double-blind randomized control cross-over trial." *European Journal of Pain* 24 (9): 1716–1729. https://doi.org/10.1002/ejp.1615

Hartescu, Iuliana, Kevin Morgan, and Clare D. Stevinson. 2015. "Increased physical activity improves sleep and mood outcomes in inactive people with insomnia: A randomized controlled trial." *Journal of Sleep Research* 24 (5):526–534. https://doi.org/10.1111/jsr.12297

Luthringer, R., M. Muzet, N. Zisapel, and L. Staner. 2009. "The effect of prolonged-release melatonin on sleep measures and psychomotor performance in elderly patients with insomnia." *International Clinical Psychopharmacology* 24 (5): 239–249. https://doi.org/10.1097/YIC.0b013e32832e9b08

Pan, Z., M. Huang, J. Huang, Z. Yao, and Z. Lin. 2020. "Association of napping and all-cause mortality and incident cardiovascular diseases: A dose-response meta analysis of cohort studies." *Sleep Medicine* 74: 165–172. https://doi.org/10.1016/j.sleep.2020.08.009

Sasseville, A., and M. Hébert. 2010. "Using blue-green light at night and blue-blockers during the day to improves adaptation to night work: a pilot study." *Progress in Neuro-Psychopharmacology & Biological Psychiatry* 34 (7): 1236–1242. https://doi.org/10.1016/j.pnpbp.2010.06.027

Wade, A. G., I. Ford, G. Crawford, A. D. McMahon, T. Nir, M. Laudon, and N. Zisapel. 2007. "Efficacy of prolonged release melatonin in insomnia patients aged 55-80 years: Quality of sleep and next-day alertness outcomes." *Current Medical Research and Opinion* 23 (10): 2597–2605. https://doi.org/10.1185/030079907X233098

RESOURCES

Government of Canada. 2019. "Are Canadian adults getting enough sleep?" https://www.canada.ca/en/public-health/services/publications/healthy-living/canadian-adults-getting-enough-sleep-infographic.html

National Sleep Foundation (United States): https://www.sleepfoundation.org/

STEP 4: FIX YOUR DIET

REFERENCES

US Department of Agriculture (USDA). 2022. *Food Security in the U.S.* https://www.ers.usda.gov/topics/food-nutrition-assistance/food-security-in-the-u-s/key-statistics-graphics/

American Heart Association. 2021. "What Is Metabolic Syndrome?" https://www.heart.org/en/health-topics/metabolic-syndrome/about-metabolic-syndrome

RESOURCES

Canada Food Guide. 2022. Information for Consumers. https://food-guide.canada.ca/en/healthy-eating-resources/

STEP 5: GET HELP FROM OTHERS

REFERENCES

Goldstein, Pavel, Irit Weissman-Fogel, Guillaume Dumas, and Simone G. Shamay-Tsoory. 2018. "Brain-to-brain coupling during handholding is associated with pain reduction." *The Proceedings of the National Academy of Sciences (PNAS)* 115 (11) E2528–E2537. https://doi.org/10.1073/pnas.1703643115

Villemure, C., and M. C. Bushnell. 2009. "Mood influences supraspinal pain processing separately from attention." *Journal of Neuroscience* 29 (3): 705–715. https://doi.org/10.1523/JNEUROSCI.3822-08.2009

Treede, Rolf-Detlef, Winfried Rief, Antonia Barke, Qasim Aziz, Michael I. Bennett, Rafael Benoliel, Milton Cohen, et al. 2019. "Chronic pain as a symptom or a disease: The IASP Classification of Chronic Pain for the International Classification of Diseases (ICD-11). *Pain* 160 (1):19–27. doi:10.1097/j.pain.0000000000001384

RESOURCES

American Chronic Pain Association: https://www.theacpa.org/

Arthritis Foundation (USA): https://www.arthritis.org/

Arthritis Society Canada: https://arthritis.ca/

Australian Pain Management Association: https://www.painmanagement.org.au/

Fibromyalgia Association of Canada: https://fibrocanada.ca/en/

Global Alliance of Partners for Pain Advocacy (International): https://www.gappa-pain.org/

Migraine Canada: https://migrainecanada.org/

Pain Canada: https://www.paincanada.ca/resources/resources-for-people-with-pain

Pain Concern (UK): https://painconcern.org.uk/

Solutions for Kids in Pain (Canada): https://kidsinpain.ca/

The Pain Toolkit UK: https://www.paintoolkit.org

The U.S. Pain Foundation: https://uspainfoundation.org/

STEP 6: CHECK YOUR MEDICINE CABINET

RESOURCES

Drug Approvals and Databases from US Food and Drug Administration (USFDA): https://www.fda.gov/drugs/development-approval-process-drugs/drug-approvals-and-databases

Drug Product Database (DPD) from Health Canada: Search the DPD to find drugs authorized for sale by Health Canada. https://www.canada.ca/en/health-canada/services/drugs-health-products/drug-products/drug-product-database.html

STEP 7: MAKE ROOM IN YOUR TOOLBOX

REFERENCES

ACSM. 2022. *ACSM's Guidelines for Exercise Testing and Prescription, 11th Edition.* Edited by Gary Liguori. American College of Sports Medicine (ACSM)

RESOURCES

Canadian Society for Exercise Physiology (CSEP): https://csepguidelines.ca/

Government of Canada. *Physical Activity Tips for Adults* (18-64 years). https://www.canada.ca/en/public-health/services/publications/healthy-living/physical-activity-tips-adults-18-64-years.html

HealthLinkBC. 2021. *Overcoming Barriers: Adding More Physical Activity to your Life.* 2021. https://www.healthlinkbc.ca/healthy-eating-physical-activity/being-active/overcoming-barriers-adding-more-physical-activity

STEP 8: FOCUS ON YOUR GOALS

RESOURCES

Hyatt, Michael, and Daniel Harkavy. 2016. *Living Forward: A Proven Plan to Stop Drifting and Get the Life You Want.* Grand Rapids, MI: Baker Publishing Group. https://livingforwardbook.com/

Library and Archives Canada Cataloguing in Publication

Title: 8 steps to conquer chronic pain : a doctor's guide to lifelong relief / Dr. Andrea Furlan, MD, PhD, PM&R.

Other titles: Eight steps to conquer chronic pain

Names: Furlan, Andrea (Andrea Dompieri), author.

Description: Includes index.

Identifiers: Canadiana 20220455880 | ISBN 9780778807117 (softcover)

Subjects: LCSH: Chronic pain—Treatment.

Classification: LCC RB127 .F87 2023 | DDC 616/.0472—dc23

INDEX

as treatment tool, 58, 224–31
MRI (magnetic resonance
  imaging), 47–48
muscles, 144, 156. *See also*
  myofascial pain syndrome
  relaxing, 207, 233–34
music therapy, 236
myofascial pain syndrome
  (MPS), 232–33

N

nabilone, 210, 214
naproxen, 153, 210
naps, 129–30
narcotics. *See* opioids
neck pain, 92, 98
neglect. *See* adverse childhood
  experiences
nerve blocks, 208
nervous system, 22–23, 32–34.
  See also brain
  parasympathetic (PNS), 26, 101
  rewiring, 67–68
  sympathetic (SNS), 26, 97, 208
neuralgia, 29, 31, 144
neuropathic. *See* pain,
  neuropathic
neurotransmitters, 116
nicotine, 106, 211–12
nocebo effect, 195
nociception, 22, 88, 90. *See also*
  pain, nociceptive
nociceptors, 22, 37, 88, 90, 160
nociplastic. *See* pain, nociplastic
nocturia, 128
nortriptyline, 205
NSAIDs, 195, 199, 210
nutrition. *See* diet; malnutrition

O

obesity, 136, 143, 146
omega-3/-6 essential fatty acids,
  153
opioids, 175–79, 200–204. *See
  also* substance-use disorder
  endogenous, 24–25, 104, 203–4,
    210
  as pain cause, 190, 201
  side effects, 195, 202
  starting, 177
  tapering, 175–76, 194, 198–99
  use of, 105, 106, 204
  withdrawal from, 199, 203–4
optimism, 82
orphenadrine, 207
osteoarthritis, 154–55, 230–31
  joint lubrication for, 94, 225,
    230, 231
osteoporosis, 150–51, 228–30
oxycodone. *See* opioids

P

pain, 20. *See also* pain
  management; *specific types of
  pain (below)*
  acute vs. chronic, 30–33
  bio-psycho-social-spiritual
    model, 161–62, 222
  catastrophizing, 52, 82, 108–9,
    224
  chronic, 29, 30–33, 52, 142–43
  describing, 42–44
  diagnosis of, 40–49, 54–55, 69
  as disease, 62–64
  emotional component, 90, 160
  equipment for dealing with, 237

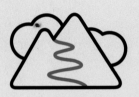